101 Tips™ for Coping with Diabetes

Richard R. Rubin, PhD, CDE
Gary Arsham, MD, PhD
Catherine Feste, BA
David G. Marrero, PhD
Stefan H. Rubin

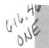

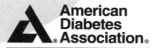

American
Diabetes
Association®

Cure • Care • Commitment℠

Director, Book Publishing, John Fedor; *Associate Director, Consumer Books,* Sherrye Landrum; *Editor,* Abe Ogden; *Production Manager,* Peggy M. Rote; *Composition,* Circle Graphics; *Cover Design,* Koncept Inc.; *Printer,* Transcontinental Printing.

Printed in Canada
3 5 7 9 10 8 6 4 2

The suggestions and information contained in this publication are generally consistent with the *Clinical Practice Recommendations* and other policies of the American Diabetes Association, but they do not represent the policy or position of the Association or any of its boards or committees. Reasonable steps have been taken to ensure the accuracy of the information presented. However, the American Diabetes Association cannot ensure the safety or efficacy of any product or service described in this publication. Individuals are advised to consult a physician or other appropriate health care professional before undertaking any diet or exercise program or taking any medication referred to in this publication. Professionals must use and apply their own professional judgment, experience, and training and should not rely solely on the information contained in this publication before prescribing any diet, exercise, or medication. The American Diabetes Association—its officers, directors, employees, volunteers, and members—assumes no responsibility or liability for personal or other injury, loss, or damage that may result from the suggestions or information in this publication.

⊚ The paper in this publication meets the requirements of the ANSI Standard Z39.48-1992 (permanence of paper).

ADA titles may be purchased for business or promotional use or for special sales. To purchase this book in large quantities, or for custom editions of this book with your logo, contact Lee Romano Sequeira, Special Sales & Promotions, at the address below, or at LRomano@diabetes.org or 703-299-2046.

American Diabetes Association
1701 North Beauregard Street
Alexandria, Virginia 22311

Library of Congress Cataloging-in-Publication Data

101 tips for coping with diabetes / Richard R. Rubin . . . [et al.].
   p. cm.
  ISBN 1-58040-143-0 (pbk. : alk. paper)
   1. Diabetes—Popular works. I. Title: One hundred and one tips for coping with diabetes.
II. Rubin, Richard R.

RC660.4 .A1453 2003
616.4'62—dc21

2002035636

CONTENTS

▼

Introduction

▼

Diabetes care today is a real good news/bad news story. On the one hand, we have so many marvelous new tools for helping people live long, healthy lives. On the other hand, few people use these tools to their full advantage. Given the countless demands of life with diabetes, it is not surprising that no one does everything right when it comes to diabetes management. Still, some people do most things right most of the time. And that usually means better blood sugar control and better physical and emotional well being; day to day and in the years to come.

People who take good care of their diabetes seem to all have one thing in common—they cope well with all the scheduled and unscheduled demands of their disease. Coping well means finding ways to maintain your glucose control and more (triglycerides, blood pressure, etc.) without sacrificing your quality of life.

The recipe for coping well includes three key ingredients: knowledge, skill, and support. You need to know how serious diabetes can be and what you can do day to day to stay healthy. You also need the skill to put that knowledge into action. Finally, you need support from your family, friends, and health care providers for the best possible health and quality of life.

This book was written to help you better cope with diabetes. It is filled with tips for increasing your diabetes knowledge, skill, and support.

The authors of this book have lots of diabetes experience. Four of them have diabetes, and the fifth has lived for over 40 years with loved ones who have diabetes. Altogether, they bring to this book almost 200 years of experience living with diabetes. We hope this experience, which we've utilized here, makes it easier to cope with your own diabetes.

The information in this book, based on the knowledge and experience of the authors, is believed to be medically accurate at the time of publication. Information and recommendations change as new information is discovered. The authors, reviewers, and publisher disclaim all liability arising from any adverse effects or results that occur or might be construed to occur as a result of the application of any of the information or recommendations in this book. If you have questions or concerns about the appropriateness or application of the information in this book, and how it may apply to you, consult your physician or other health care professional. The information in this book is not intended to replace advice from a health professional specifically tailored to you as an individual, but rather to complement it.

Chapter 1
MANAGING STRESS AND NOURISHING YOUR SOUL

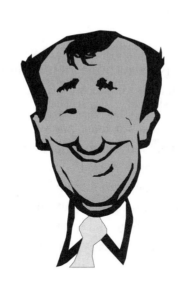

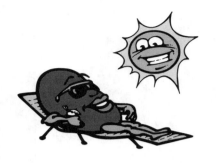

Is it okay to take a vacation from diabetes when I take my summer vacation at the beach?

▼
TIP:

Everyone needs vacations—even from diabetes. Trouble is, it's hard to take one. When you're on vacation you want to enjoy yourself as much as possible. To do that you have to feel good, and to feel good you can't take a complete vacation from your diabetes. However, you can probably take a more relaxed approach to at least some parts of your normal routine.

Think about one or two things you do to manage your diabetes that you would most like a vacation from. Things like monitoring your blood glucose, getting up early in the morning to take your insulin, or eating carefully. Are there ways you could take a vacation from these responsibilities—at least once in a while—without losing control of your diabetes? Are there adjustments you could make that allow you to miss a glucose check here and there, sleep in a little extra, or work in foods that aren't a normal part of your diet?

You are only human, and it is vacation. You need it and deserve it. There's plenty of time to get back on track later. Talk to your diabetes care team about changes you can make to your routine that can help vacation be a little more relaxing.

Can stress affect my blood glucose levels?

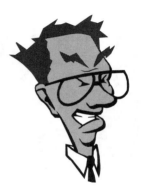

▼
TIP:

It sure can. Stress can affect your blood glucose in 2 ways. First, some people find that stress has an immediate effect on their blood sugars. Most people who notice an effect say that stress pushes their blood sugars up, but a few say that stress has the opposite effect.

Second, stress can also have a long-term "wear and tear" effect on blood glucose. Most people who have diabetes experience this effect, at least from time to time. When people feel stressed they often stop taking good care of themselves, because they are overwhelmed and don't have the energy. Ultimately, stress can trigger a negative spiral of feeling overwhelmed, doing less to manage diabetes, and having higher blood glucose levels.

Finding ways to cope with stress can help your body and your soul.

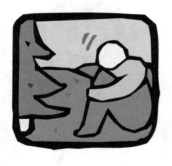

*H*ow can I keep going when nothing I do to control my diabetes seems to work?

*F*irst, make sure your goals are realistic. Perfect diabetes control is impossible, so if this is your goal, you'll probably be disappointed. You'll also be disappointed if you set goals that are personally unrealistic. Some people can run 6 miles every day, but you may not be one of them. If not, don't make that level of activity part of your diabetes management plan.

Naturally, there are times when even the most realistic goals aren't met. That's the time to remind yourself why you set the goal in the first place. If that reason still holds, it could help you get back on track. You can also think of one step, no matter how small, you could take to get you immediately on the path toward your goal. Sometimes just realizing it's possible to take a positive step can really help. And remember; if all else fails to rally your spirits, call on a family member, friend, or health care provider for the support you need.

Talk "sense" to yourself. Give yourself affirming messages for all that you're doing to manage your diabetes. Then, focus on healthy living and enjoying life. Let life be your focus, not diabetes. Remember what former American Diabetes Association (ADA) president Dr. Fred Whitehouse so wisely said, "Manage your diabetes to live; don't live to manage your diabetes."

*C*an stress management help my
diabetes?

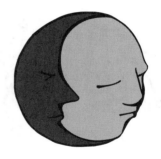

▼
TIP:

I̲t could. Everybody's life is stressful, so doing things that help you
relax is always good. Relaxing and managing your stress can also
help you control your blood glucose, since uncontrolled stress can
throw glucose levels out of whack.

There are lots of ways to relax. Think about what works for you.
How about a nice soak in a warm tub? Or a quiet time reading your
favorite magazine? Or talking on the phone to a good friend? How
about gardening or attending religious services? Some people do
formal meditation exercises or yoga or other physical activities to
relax. All of these are wonderful ways to control stress.

Diabetes adds stress to your life. Finding ways to relieve stress
can help you feel better and more able to manage your diabetes.

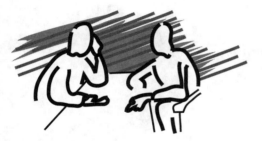

Where can I find people to talk to about living with diabetes? My family doesn't seem to get it.

▼
TIP:

Some hospitals offer educational programs and support groups for people who have diabetes. You could ask a family member to join you at a class or meeting, if you think that would be helpful. In some areas, the American Diabetes Association sponsors similar activities. Dial 1-800-DIABETES (342-2383) and ask them what they offer and where programs are held. Your health care provider may also be able to put you in touch with other people who have diabetes.

You might also try the Internet for a "virtual" support group. The ADA website, *www.diabetes.org*, is a good place to start. Be aware that what other people say on the Internet ranges from brilliant to bunk, so be sure to check out anything you see online with someone you trust before giving it a shot yourself. The ADA also publishes a wide variety of materials to help you, including *Diabetes Forecast*, and books like this one with tips for living better with diabetes.

*H*ow can I deal with the
discouragement I feel when
I don't get the results I want?

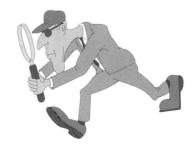

▼
TIP:

First, be sure your expectations are realistic; unrealistic expectations almost guarantee disappointment. If your goals are realistic, problem solving can boost your self-confidence and, thus, lift you out of discouragement.

The basic, time-honored process of problem solving has four steps:

1. Identify and define your problem.
2. List possible solutions.
3. Select and act on the most promising option.
4. Evaluate the outcome and keep going on your list of solutions until you feel the problem is solved.

Keep in mind the resources you have to help you problem solve. Your health care team is a good source of practical suggestions, having worked with many people who live with diabetes. Finally, by talking positively to yourself you can alleviate the stressful feelings of discouragement. Thomas Edison considered every failed experiment not as a failure, but as a lesson in what didn't work.

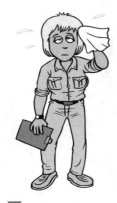

*C*an stress cause type 2 diabetes?

▼
TIP:

After lots of studies and research, the best we can say is maybe. Stress can elevate blood glucose levels. Sometimes this is the direct effect of stress hormones. Other times, it's because stress leads people to eat more and be less active, which can also raise blood glucose levels. We know this is true for people who already have diabetes. So, it seems likely that if you're blood glucose levels are already higher than normal (but not yet high enough to call it diabetes), stress could push your levels into the diabetes range.

So the stress of a serious life event, such as the death of a loved one or the loss of a job, could play a part in developing diabetes. However, it is likely you would have eventually developed diabetes anyway as insulin resistance increased or insulin production decreased.

*H*ow can I tell if I am depressed?

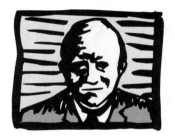

▼
TIP:

*B*eing sad is normal. Just because you're sad, doesn't mean you're "depressed." Generally, if for at least two weeks you have been feeling really sad almost all day long, or you have lost interest in most things you used to enjoy, you could be suffering from depression.

Other signs of depression include:

- Feeling bad about yourself
- Trouble concentrating and making decisions
- Feeling hopeless
- Thoughts of dying
- Trouble sleeping
- Big changes in appetite and weight

People with diabetes are much more likely to be depressed, and the consequences of this can be especially severe—depression can make it much harder to manage your diabetes. So talk to your health care provider. There are treatments for depression that work for people with diabetes.

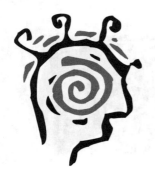 *W*hat should I do if I think I am depressed?

First, talk to your health care provider. Tell your provider that you think you might be depressed. Your health care provider can help determine whether or not this is true, or refer you to a mental health professional for diagnosis and treatment.

The good news is that there is effective treatment. Research shows that both counseling, especially a form of counseling called cognitive behavioral therapy, and antidepressant pills work to relieve depression in most people who have diabetes. Not only that, people in these studies whose depression was resolved also had closer-to-normal blood glucose levels.

So if you think you are depressed, trust your feelings and seek some assistance. Treatment can make your life happier, and healthier as well.

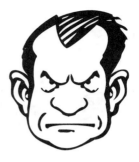

*C*ould the fact that I was diagnosed
with diabetes a few months ago be
the reason I feel angry all the time?

▼
TIP:

Maybe. Your life has changed a lot over the past few months, and it has changed in ways you didn't choose. It is normal and natural to feel angry about that. Your anger is even more understandable if your life was already pretty stressful before you developed diabetes.

Unfortunately, understandable as your anger may be, it can hurt you. Anger can burn you up and it can burn you out. Anger can push people away and cost you important support at a time when you really need it. Anger can increase your risk of having a heart attack or stroke, the leading causes of death for people with diabetes. And anger can sap your motivation for diabetes self-care. Some people even say that their blood glucose levels shoot up right away when they get angry.

So finding ways to deal with your normal, natural anger could really help.

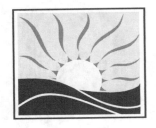

How can I find a positive way to look at diabetes management?

▼
TIP:

The real goal in diabetes management is quality of life. While diabetes management is measured by the amount of sugar in your blood, quality of life is measured by spiritual qualities like joy, peace, and love.

Inspiring stories are a source of nourishment. Stories like the poor shepherd boy, David, taking on a foe like Goliath, the giant, can inspire people to believe that they can "take on" the challenge of diabetes with the same faith as David.

Metaphor is a great way to see an old or negative situation with a new and more positive viewpoint. The author Louisa May Alcott said: "I am not afraid of storms, for I am learning how to sail my ship." Like sailing, diabetes management requires specific skills. To sail our ships successfully we need to know how to manage the physical aspects of diabetes. Equally important is the psychological, social, and spiritual stamina that helps us to cope with diabetes and any other storm that life presents. As captain of your ship, you need to make sure that you have access to resources that can provide physical, mental, and spiritual ballast.

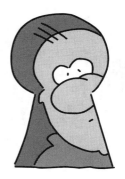

Why do I feel anxious all the time?

Lots of people feel anxious, whether they have diabetes or not, especially these days. Having diabetes only adds to the burden of worry. It can be hard to tell the difference between normal, and even useful, worrying and the kind that indicates a problem.

If you feel anxious all or almost all the time, it is probably a problem. Try to picture as clearly and specifically as you can what worries you. Picture it and describe it to yourself in detail. Does anything help you manage your worry? If so, how can you more often do what helps? If nothing helps and you can't think of anything that would help, talk to your health care provider for suggestions.

Low blood glucose levels can also contribute to anxiety. When people are low, they often say they feel shaky and agitated, and since low blood glucose can be embarrassing and even dangerous, many people worry a lot about getting low. In a sense, you can get anxious about low glucose anxieties. Preventing lows is important, but so is preventing highs, so you want to deal realistically with your anxiety about low blood glucose.

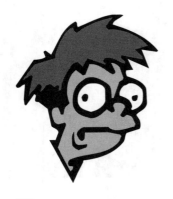

I've just been diagnosed with type 2 diabetes and it all seems very overwhelming. How can I make all the changes I'm supposed to make?

▼
TIP:

First, remember that you do not have to do everything at once. There are lots of changes to make, but they don't need to be made overnight. Also keep in mind that you are not alone in this. People who want to help you, including your health care team, family, and friends, are all around you. Make sure you draw on these resources to help you make needed changes. In addition to the support, you need the following three things to make changes:

- Knowledge (about your diabetes)
- Motivation (a reason to change that means a lot to you)
- Resources (health care providers, family, personal strengths)

You can learn more about your diabetes by talking to your health care provider or participating in a diabetes education program at the local hospital. Call the American Diabetes Association at 1-800-DIABETES or visit *www.diabetes.org*. Having a reason to change is so important. Take time to be clear in your own mind and heart why you want to make changes. Then you can remind yourself later, when your commitment may be wavering. Resources to help you change are everywhere, and they can be very helpful once you are committed to making a change.

M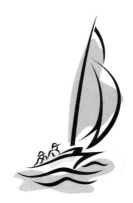*aking changes to manage my diabetes is so hard. How can I make it easier?*

▼
TIP:

By making your changes more tangible. Consider a change you've been thinking of making. Pick a specific thing you want to do differently. Ask yourself, on a scale of 1 to 5, how important that change is to you. Next, ask yourself, on a scale of 1 to 5, how confident you are that you can make this change. Reflect on the barriers you may encounter as you attempt to reach your goal, and how you would overcome those barriers. Have you ever failed at an attempt to overcome this behavior? What's different about this time? Why are you confident that you will succeed?

As you list your reasons for success, list the rewards—both internal (like the pleasure of knowing you have succeeded) and concrete (like buying yourself a new article of clothing, a book, tickets to an event). Continue asking yourself the questions:

- How important is this to me?
- How confident am I that I can do it?

And, never give up. A German proverb says: "Patience is a bitter plant, but it has sweet fruit."

Chapter 2
EATING HEALTHIER AND CONTROLLING YOUR WEIGHT

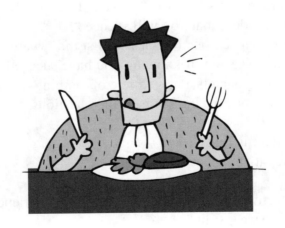

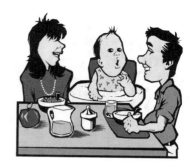

I know I need to eat healthier because I have diabetes. How can I get my family to stop insisting I cook meals with lots of fat and sugar?

▼
TIP:

Try to strike a compromise with your family. For every time you cook a "rich" meal, they have to eat a meal low in fat and sugar. You can work out the most agreeable trade-off.

Also, you can probably make switches to cut "hidden" fat and sugar, like salsa on your potato, and skim milk instead of whole. Check out the many wonderful cookbooks that the American Diabetes Association has published. There are lots of great tips for cooking low fat and keeping carbs under control.

If you and your family have been accustomed to meals that are high in fat and sugar, you may want to make changes as slowly as possible. Instead of a high-fat salad, high-fat entrée, and a high-fat, high-sugar dessert, substitute a healthier item for one of the high-fat dishes. At another meal make a similar change with another dish. Slow changes will be more acceptable to your family and are more likely to stick. You can even avoid telling your family you've made the switch to healthier fare. They may not notice!

As you know, a diet that's good for people with diabetes is good for everyone. You're not helping just yourself, you're helping your whole family.

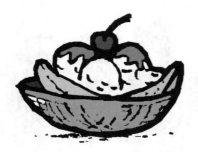

How do I deal with the temptation of desserts when I eat at other people's houses?

Offer to bring the dessert. Make something you really like that your family and friends enjoy as well. Most people are happy to have a guest to bring some part of the meal.

And remember, you can work in dessert. Tips for successfully "working in" dessert include:

- Skipping another part of the meal, like bread or potato
- Having a small portion. Sometimes a few mouthfuls will satisfy your craving
- Extending enjoyment by eating slowly, savoring the flavor
- Doing some activity after eating
- Monitoring blood glucose an hour or two after eating to see what adjustments are called for

*H*ow can I stick to a meal plan when my schedule at work is so unpredictable?

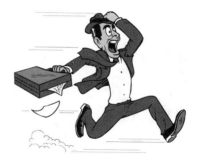

▼
TIP:

*E*ating something as close to your normal eating times as possible can help. Try carrying easy-to-eat foods with you, such as trail mix or carrots. That way you can satisfy your hunger without pushing your blood sugars too high. You can also check your blood glucose before you eat a snack or meal. If your blood sugar is on the high side, you don't need to eat unless you're hungry.

If you eat a snack to tide you over, try to eat a little less at your next meal. Focus on eating reasonable servings and avoiding large amounts of sweets. Finally, if you find yourself eating at an odd time, try to work in some exercise after your meal to help burn off a few of the calories and keep your blood glucose level closer to normal.

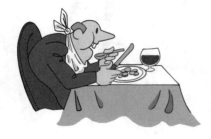

I find it hard to stay on my diet, and whenever I splurge I feel so guilty that I just keep on splurging for days. What can I do?

▼
TIP:

It was once said that the best way to deal with a temptation is to yield to it! Staying on a diet forever is extremely hard. So the first step is to recognize that *everyone* splurges. It's natural, normal, and even inevitable. If you accept this and it helps you feel less guilty, you might be able to splurge in a more controlled way.

You can also try the "3-to-1 rule." The 3-to-1 rule is as follows: Each time you indulge in a food splurge, follow it with 3 equal units of time in which you eat a more sensible, predictable diet. The time period in question can vary. It could be a single meal, a day, even a weekend. For example, if you eat voraciously for a day, eat conservatively for the following three days. Remember, good diabetes control is a game of averages, not a game of perfection!

I cannot control my eating in the evening between dinner and bedtime. What should I do?

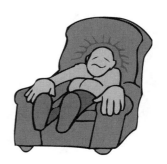

▼
TIP:

Get busy! Distract yourself from thinking about food by getting involved in an activity that so absorbs you, food doesn't even make it to your radar screen. Some people report that leaving the house is helpful. You could take a walk, do an errand, or visit a friend (and let your friend know what you're doing so that you're not offered snacks). If you are at home, clean a closet, do wood-working, play the piano, or read a book that you know will completely absorb you. Make a list of a few projects, so if you finish one you have another to start.

Make a decision (even a formal contract with yourself) about the times you absolutely will not eat, like when you're reading or watching television. Tell yourself that you will eat only while sitting at the kitchen or dining room table and only during meal times or scheduled snack times.

Another winning technique is to avoid overstocking the refrigerator and pantry. If there is not much food available, it is much easier to avoid eating between meals.

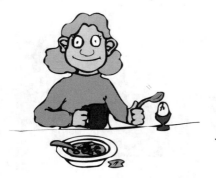

I'm shocked by how high my blood sugar is after a meal. Would eating smaller meals more frequently help?

▼
TIP:

It could help. Though this approach is not for everyone, it does have advantages for many people with diabetes, including:

- Lower blood glucose levels after eating (because less food is eaten)
- Lower total insulin needs for those who take insulin
- Lower cholesterol levels
- Less hunger, so fewer calories are consumed throughout the day

There are some diabetes pills, such as acarbose (Precose) and miglitol (Glyset), that slow the absorption of food and have similar effects to eating smaller meals.

For more, talk to your health care provider about this approach to keeping your blood glucose level closer to normal throughout the day.

101 Tips for Coping with Diabetes

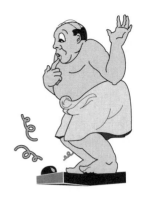

I'm struggling to control my weight. Should I see a dietitian?

▼
TIP:

EVERYONE who has diabetes should see a registered dietitian (RD). There are three very important reasons for this:

1. **Diabetes management** is greatly dependent upon the type of food you eat and the amount of food you eat.
2. **Good nutrition** is a basic and important part of a healthy life. A dietitian will recommend a meal plan that contains nutritionally well-balanced food and good taste.
3. A dietitian can help you with **weight management**, an important goal for most people with diabetes.

Weight management means taking in less energy (calories) than you put out (activity). That's a good way to remember that activity is an important part of weight control.

Both the American Dietetic Association (1-800-877-1600 ext. 5000, or *www.eatright.org/find.html*) and the American Association of Diabetes Educators (1-800-TEAM-UP-4, or *www.aadenet.org*) have hotlines and websites that can give you the names of dietitians in your area.

I almost always feel stuffed (and guilty) after eating at a restaurant. What can I do?

▼
TIP:

This can be very difficult. Restaurants today serve almost criminal amounts of food as a single meal. Cleaning your plate usually means you've eaten enough food for three people. Therefore, portion control is very important. The following tips should help you keep your food intake at a reasonable level.

- First, become a taster. If you're dining with friends who like to share, trading tastes can add variety, and variety can help make up for quantity.
- Second, when you are served your main course, divide the portions (meat, vegetables, starch) in half, and ask the server to put your "leftovers" in a bag to take home for later. This will leave you feeling comfortably full rather than stuffed, and it means you'll have another delicious meal the next night.
- Finally, tune in to your body. Pay attention to how you feel when you are getting full. Learn to stop eating when you feel this way, even if your plate is not empty.

101 Tips for Coping with Diabetes

I *know I should be counting carbs*
to improve my blood sugar control,
but I'm having trouble learning how.
Where should I turn for help?

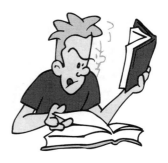

▼
TIP:

Talk with a registered dietitian who can help you figure it out.
There is usually one associated with your local hospital. If this
is not a good solution for you, look for an Internet site with carb
counting help. For example, you could try using the carb counting
flash card deck made by Carb Cards (*www.carbcards.com*). Each
card has an image and the name of a type of food on it, along with
the carbohydrate count for each item. You can combine the cards to
build a food pyramid and create daily menus. Sometimes a picture is
worth a thousand words!

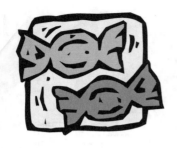

Is it okay to eat candy? I love it and don't want to give it up.

It is okay to eat anything as long as you don't eat too much and you know how much you're eating, so you can make adjustments to keep your blood glucose close to normal. More and more candy and sweets have labels with a nutritional analysis, including the amount of carbohydrate and fat, so it is easier to know how much you are eating. When you know that, you can compensate by eating less of something else, exercising, or taking more insulin (if this is an option).

Some people eat their favorite candy to treat low blood sugar. The challenge here can be controlling the number you eat, especially if you really like the candy and you're so low you aren't thinking clearly.

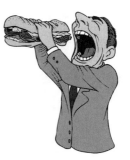

I'm confused about what I am supposed to eat. What is a healthy diet for people with diabetes?

TIP:

The same diet that is healthy for everyone—one that includes grains, beans, fruits, vegetables, low-fat dairy products, and meats. You don't need special foods because of diabetes, but you should do what you can to cut back on foods with lots of fat (like lunch meats, salad dressings, cheeses, and fried foods), lots of added sugar (like soft drinks), or both (like desserts and candies).

If you are taking insulin or other diabetes medication, the timing of your meals could also be important for keeping your blood glucose levels as close to normal as possible throughout the day. Keeping track of how different foods affect your blood glucose can also help you choose a healthy meal plan.

Seeing a registered dietitian (RD) can make this process easier and more effective. An RD can work with you to see what type of foods you like, what you don't like, and what would work best for your diabetes management. Together, you can come up with a meal plan that works for you.

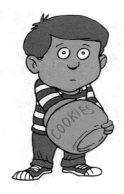

*S*ometimes I can't stop eating. Is this
because of my diabetes?

▼
TIP:

It could be. There are many reasons why people can't stop eating.
Sometimes it is more mental than physical. Since eating provides
an immediate satisfaction, some people eat to cope with emotional
needs that have little to do with physical hunger. And because eating
doesn't truly satisfy these needs, these feelings often return very
quickly and the person will keep eating. If diabetes makes your life
feel less satisfying, it could contribute to your problem.

Another group of people physically can't tell when they've eaten
enough. For some reason or another, their bodies don't signal that
they're full and they continue to eat long after they've eaten more
than they need.

Still other people eat to protect themselves from low blood
glucose. Some are so afraid of ever going low that they constantly
keep their levels really high. Dealing with these natural fears can
make a big difference. People who frequently go low need to adjust
their diabetes management plan, not overeat. Talk to your health
care provider about any issues that might be causing your
overeating.

Chapter 3
BEING MORE ACTIVE

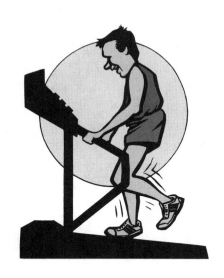

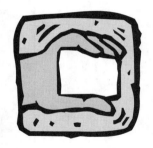

I *don't like to carry things in my hands while I'm active, so it's a hassle to carry a fast acting carb with me while I exercise. What can I do?*

▼
TIP:

There are a few solutions to this problem.

■ First, try carrying a fanny pack with a few carbs and perhaps a small glucose meter. Several companies make packs designed for athletes.

■ You could also try carrying a couple of small tubes of cake icing in some wristbands. They are light, resistant to sweat and moisture, and contain a very concentrated form of glucose.

■ Some athletes with diabetes actually place a roll of LifeSavers inside the webbing of their shoelaces. This doesn't add much weight and by being placed inside your shoelaces, you're not as likely to nibble on them randomly.

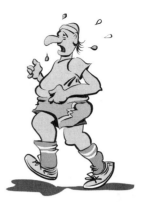

I *worry that I will go low while*
exercising. How do I adjust my insulin so
this doesn't happen?

TIP:

Figuring out the best adjustment can take a bit of trial and error. First, ask your health care provider for advice. Second, do what serious and professional athletes do: Keep a training log. In your training log, you'll want to record the following things:

- Type of exercise
- Time of exercise
- Duration and intensity of your session
- What you eat before you start
- Most importantly, your blood glucose before you start and after you stop exercising

Since exercise can cause you to continue using glucose after you stop your session, it is important to measure your glucose about one hour after your session ends. By reviewing your training log, you will be able to see what did and did not work for you.

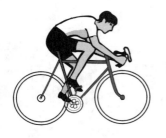

I don't want to run out of energy while I'm exercising. What should I eat to prevent this?

What foods you use depends on 3 things—the type of exercise you are doing, the duration and intensity, and your blood glucose level before exercising. If your blood glucose is below 150 mg/dl before you exercise, it is probably a good idea to eat about 15 grams of carbohydrate. This could be a serving of starch, fruit, or milk. You might also consider using foods that you really like, but usually don't eat because they have a negative impact on your blood sugars. One athlete we know enjoys eating a Snickers bar before his workouts. As he says, "I know there are better sources of energy, such as sports drinks, but I really like Snickers. So the way I see it, if I need to scratch my chocolate itch, I might as well do it when I know that the exercise will burn up most of the glucose!"

*H*ow can I exercise regularly when I work all day?

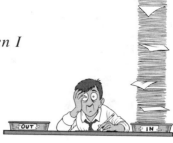

▼

TIP:

*F*irst of all, remember that *exercise* really means *activity*, so lots of things you don't consider to be exercise actually are. Just as important, you don't have to be active for large blocks of time to reap the benefits. Several short "bursts" of activity in a day can be just as good for you.

Try to make the most of opportunities to be active during the normal course of your day. Take the stairs instead of the elevator. Park at the far end of the parking lot and walk to the store. Set aside 10 minutes of your lunchtime for a brisk walk. You may be pleasantly surprised with your total daily activity level if you take advantage of opportunities like these.

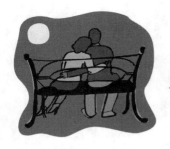

*H*ow *many calories do I burn when my wife and I are intimate?*

▼ TIP:

*S*ex is exercise, just like running or swimming. Like all exercise, the number of calories you burn making love depends on the duration and intensity of the activity, as well as your weight (the more you weigh, the more calories you burn doing the same activity). The average caloric consumption during lovemaking has been calculated at 250 calories an hour.

If your blood glucose tends to go low during sex or immediately after, you might want to check your level just before or after you make love. If you are low or headed in that direction, it's best to eat something. This can briefly interrupt your loving interlude, but it can also help prevent the more serious interruption of a low glucose episode.

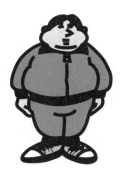

*W*hat can you suggest for a person who
really dislikes exercise?

▼ TIP:

First, we will remove the word *exercise*. Researchers have found that you don't really need to exercise. Just any old kind of physical activity is good enough, if you do it regularly. As little as 30 minutes of moderate activity (like brisk walking) a day can do you good. Try to find an activity that you actually like doing. The possibilities are endless—walking the dog, swimming, dancing or even playing with a child or grandchild.

Try to pair that activity with something else you like to do. For example, if you regularly talk to a friend on the phone or over the back fence, go for a walk with that person instead. Or, if it's feasible to walk to work or the store instead of taking the bus or driving, give that a try.

You can also set some activity goals or milestones, and reward yourself as you progress and reach them. You decide on the reward. Eventually, you may find you are feeling better and are actually enjoying the activity, and the activity itself becomes its own reward.

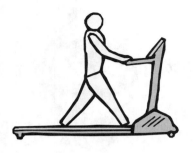

Is it safe to exercise if I have heart problems?

▼
TIP:

If you have heart problems, the American Diabetes Association recommends you have an exercise stress test before you start exercising. An exercise stress test shows how a workout affects your heart and blood pressure. The test also helps to detect "silent" heart disease (heart disease that has no symptoms), which is more common in people who have diabetes.

During an exercise stress test, you walk on a treadmill while your heart function and blood pressure are monitored. You start at a slow pace and gradually build up until you get tired or something unusual shows up on the monitor. The test usually lasts a few minutes and rarely lasts longer than 20 minutes. After the test is done, the doctor who did the test will tell you about the results, including any problems that need treatment and any conditions you need to take into account when you exercise.

*W*here can I find someone to walk with?

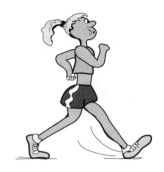

▼
TIP:

Many people find it easier to exercise when they have company. Start by asking people you know who might be willing to join you. Check with family members, friends, and co-workers. Try to find someone dependable who is at about your level of fitness. If no one you know is interested or available, see if any of the malls in your area has a walking program, or look in your local paper for walking clubs. Almost all cities have several, for all ages and levels of fitness. Walking clubs are fun and the members are always happy to have you join them. You could also start walking at the track at a local school; you are almost certain to find other walkers there. Seek and you shall find.

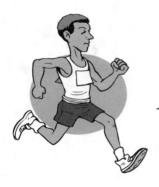

I want to compete in a 5-k run. What should I do to prepare?

Competing can be fun and rewarding, as long as you stay safe. First, check with your health care provider to be sure that you're physically able to train for competition. Once you've been checked out, be sure your goals for the run are realistic. Your first goal should be to have fun, and your second should be to finish the run feeling good. Try to keep your time for the race lower on your list of priorities.

Next, you have to train so you will be ready to reach your goals. A healthy goal is to build up your weekly training mileage to between 10–15 miles a week. Start with runs of a mile or less and work up to 3 miles or a little longer (5 kilometers is about 3.1 miles). By the time of the race you should be able to run 5 km comfortably. Don't worry about the speed of your training runs. If you want to get some idea of what your race-day time will be, about 2–3 weeks before the race run 5 km as fast as you comfortably can and time yourself. You will probably run a bit faster on race day because your adrenaline will be flowing.

*C*an exercise cause my blood glucose
to drop hours later?

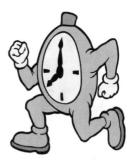

▼

TIP:

Yes. Depending on the intensity and duration of your activity,
you can burn glucose for up to 24 hours after exercise. With
long or hard exercise, you use sugars stored in your liver for fuel.
After the exercise is over, your body wants to replenish those sugars
as soon as possible. If there is no food available, the sugars are
pulled from your blood stream, which can cause hypoglycemia.
To help prevent low blood glucose, check your blood sugar about
every 45 minutes after a hard workout and gauge whether your
blood sugar is going down, going up, or leveling off. If it is going
down, eat a few carbs and keep checking until you level off.

*I*s it safe to exercise if my blood glucose is high?

This depends on how high and how much insulin you have on board. If your blood glucose is higher than 300 mg/dl, you should not exercise until you have taken some fast-acting insulin and your blood glucose level is below 250 mg/dl. The problem is this: If your glucose is high and you don't have enough insulin in your body to use the glucose, your cells will continue to signal they need glucose for fuel, and your liver will continue to put out that glucose. Without insulin to let the glucose into the cells, the glucose keeps building up in your blood, pushing your blood glucose levels higher and higher.

If you have enough insulin available, exercise may actually help lower your glucose. In fact, many athletes raise their blood sugar before exercise on purpose to create a bit of a buffer so they won't go low during their activity.

*H*ow can I exercise if I don't get around very well?

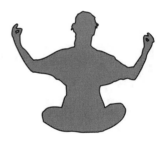

▼
TIP:

There are activities for everyone. Swimming or water aerobics are easy on your body, and there are chair exercises you can do sitting down. You can also try yoga or tai chi for no-impact exercise. Some of these activities require equipment (like a swimming pool), or some training (like yoga or tai chi), but others (like chair exercises) can be done anywhere at all with "equipment" you already have at home.

Try lifting cans of food while sitting in a chair watching television, or try waving around dishcloths while listening to music to increase your range of motion and your fitness. There are also books and videotapes on exercise available for people who have limited mobility. So look for ways to increase your activity despite your limitations. You will be glad you did.

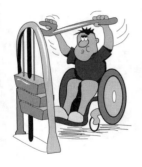

It's hard for me to get motivated about exercising. Will buying exercise equipment help me exercise more regularly?

▼
TIP:

It could, if you find something you really like. On the other hand, you don't want to spend lots of money on something that ends up being an expensive clothes rack. There are 3 keys to finding the right exercise equipment for you.

- First, decide on your activity goals. If you want to walk, the only equipment you'll need is a good pair of shoes and comfortable clothes. Strength training will require some free weights or a piece of equipment, perhaps one that lets you do a variety of exercises.
- Second, think about your space and money limitations. These will determine what, if any, equipment it makes sense to consider.
- Finally, try before you buy, especially if you're thinking about spending a lot of money. If you think a particular piece of equipment might be right for you, try it out at a friend's house, at the store, or at a local health club.

The right equipment can really help you stay active, so make sure the one you buy is the right one for you.

101 Tips for Coping with Diabetes

Starting an exercise program isn't a problem. How do I stick with it?

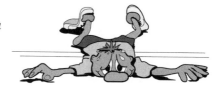

▼
TIP:

You're in the same boat as a lot of people we know. Activity is like weight loss. Most people who want to lose weight have succeeded, often many times. But the trick is not losing weight— it's keeping it off.

Here are some keys to sticking with an activity program:

- Pick only things you like to do (or at least things you don't hate to do).
- Pick more than one activity (to avoid boredom, deal with weather problems, and cross-train).
- Be realistic. Don't expect to do what you could when you were in high school.
- Get company for your activity (to add to your motivation and pleasure).
- Make appointments with yourself to exercise (to help you stay on schedule).
- Reward yourself. Staying active is a major accomplishment, so regularly reward yourself for your effort.

Chapter 4
KEEPING BLOOD GLUCOSE LEVELS CLOSER TO NORMAL

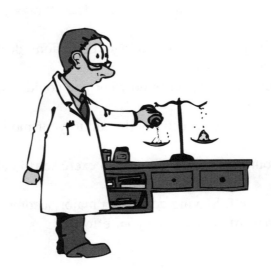

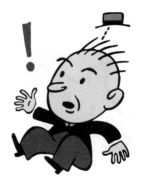

*H*ow can I do the same thing everyday for a week and then suddenly get a blood glucose reading that is totally out of whack?

▼
TIP:

It would be wonderful if there were a precise formula for keeping blood glucose levels right where you want them; this much food, this much activity, and this much medication, and your blood glucose is always in range. But it doesn't work that way. No 2 days are exactly the same, so controlling diabetes requires constant monitoring and adjustment. Often, just when you think you have a plan that works reliably, something shifts; sometimes it's things you can't control or things you may not even recognize. Understanding yourself and the way you feel is the best tool for constant and complete management. If you know when your blood glucose is heading high or low—which takes regular monitoring—you can act on these ups and downs, and maximize your time spent in that lovely "normal" range.

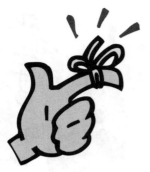

I have trouble getting blood out of my finger. Are there ways to make it easier?

Before lancing your finger:

- Wash it in warm water to get the blood flowing.
- Shake your finger down like a thermometer.
- Milk your finger.
- Put a rubber band around your finger just tight enough to make the tip of your finger red. Remove the rubber band as soon as you draw blood.

Also consider these suggestions:

- If no blood appears after you lance, wait about 5 seconds before squeezing. This gives the blood enough time to surface. If you squeeze too soon, you can sometimes have the opposite effect and decrease the flow.
- Try lancets of different lengths to find the one that works best for you.
- Try one of the alternate-site monitors to draw blood from your hands and arms.

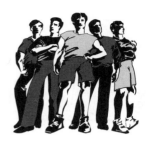

I *hate checking my blood glucose in* *public. What can I do?*

▼
TIP:

Your feelings are natural. Your diabetes is your business and it should not be anyone else's unless you want it to be. However, finding a private place to check your glucose can be difficult. Look for a quiet corner, or even a restroom stall if that is the only private place you can find. However, you may be surprised how few people even notice when you check your blood in public.

Some of the new blood glucose monitors are smaller, quicker, and quieter, and that can help make the process less stressful. Finally, if there is no place at all where you would be comfortable checking your glucose while you are out, check just before you leave the house, and check again as soon as you get home. That way you'll have at least some information for making decisions while you are out.

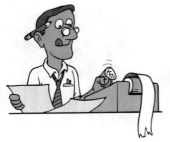

How can I afford to check my blood glucose as often as I should?

▼
TIP:

Monitoring your blood glucose can be expensive. The strips you use to check twice a day can cost as much as $700 a year. If you don't have good health insurance, you may have to pay all of that yourself. If you are having trouble paying for your strips, talk to your health care provider. Your provider could help you find a source for limited supplies of free strips, a less expensive strip to use, or different insurance plans that have better reimbursement for strips. You can also make the most of information you get from limited monitoring by checking at different times each day. For example, check before and after your breakfast one day, before and after lunch the next, etc. Remember, some information is always better than none at all. Talk to your health care provider to decide on the best monitoring schedule for you.

I *don't like to carry my insulin* *and a syringe with me when* *I'm away from home. What should* *I do?*

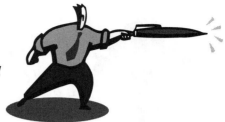

▼
TIP:

Fortunately, there are alternatives to a vial and syringe. One of our favorites is an insulin pen. An insulin pen is a small device that looks like a large fountain pen and enables you to easily take your insulin away from home—you just dial the dose you need. They are small, discreet, and protect your insulin vial from breaking. Insulin pens are the most popular way to deliver insulin in most other countries of the world, but they are just beginning to catch on in the United States. Your health care provider can tell you more about insulin pens and show you your options.

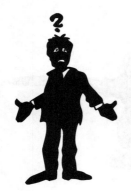

I *have type 1 diabetes, use an insulin pump,*
and lead a pretty stable life. Do I really
have to check my blood glucose 4-8 times
a day?

▼
TIP:

Not necessarily. However, be sure to talk with your health care provider before changing your glucose monitoring schedule. The safest days to reduce checks are very predictable ones, when your blood glucose before breakfast is close to normal. Take your normal boluses for any food you eat and pay close attention to any signs your blood glucose might be too high or too low. Check your level if you are not sure.

If your food or activity varies from usual, you should check more frequently. Finally, it's always wise to check your glucose before bed, just to confirm that the day has gone as expected, blood-sugar-wise.

My doctor wants me to check my glucose more frequently, but it's always a hassle. Half the time I can't find my meter, and even when I know where it is, it's usually not where I am. What can I do?

TIP:

No one enjoys checking blood glucose. Different people dislike it for different reasons. If for you it's the fact your monitor is never where you are, getting extra monitors could help. Monitors are often provided free or at very low cost, because the companies that make monitors make their money on test strips, not the monitors themselves. So you might be able to get an extra monitor or two pretty cheaply. Keep the monitors where you are most likely to be using them. For example, keep one by your bed (good for testing when you get up or go to bed), keep another in your kitchen (good for testing before meals), and keep another where you work. If you work out of your car, be careful of extreme temperatures, both for your monitor and your strips. Do not keep them in the glove box or trunk, and carry them with you if it is very hot or very cold.

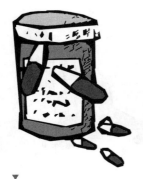

I'm taking several new diabetes medications and don't really understand what they are and how they work. How can I learn more?

▼
TIP:

There are lots of new diabetes medications available, and the number is growing rapidly. So it makes sense to stay informed about ones that might be right for you. New insulins are being introduced all the time, and we now have diabetes pills to help you control your blood glucose levels in different ways. There are pills that help you make more insulin, pills that control the release of glucose from your liver into your blood, pills that help your body use insulin better, and pills that slow the absorption of food. Since different medications help control glucose in different ways, many people take two or more diabetes pills to get the most benefit. Your health care provider is your best source of information about new diabetes medications, because your provider knows you and your diabetes.

You can find information on new diabetes medications from other places as well, including publications of the American Diabetes Association, such as *Diabetes Forecast*, and on the ADA website (*www.diabetes.org*). Many pharmaceutical companies also maintain websites with information about their new products.

My doctor wants me to start taking insulin, but when my mother started taking it years ago she developed complications. Will that happen to me?

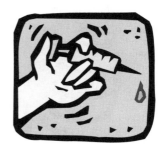

▼
TIP:

No. We can't promise you won't get complications if you take insulin, but we can assure you that insulin itself does not cause complications. In fact, taking insulin will actually *reduce* your risk of getting complications. That's because complications are the result of having high blood glucose for a long time, and insulin can help *lower* blood glucose. So insulin usually cuts your risk of complications; it doesn't increase it.

You mention that your mother developed complications after she started taking insulin, but the insulin is almost certainly not to blame. Since complications are the result of years of high blood glucose, the truth is this: your mother would almost certainly have developed complications if she had not started taking insulin, and the complications would have come sooner and been more severe. Please don't let your concerns compromise your health. If you take insulin when you need it, you can help prevent complications, not cause them.

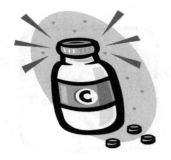

I'm looking for anything that might lower my blood sugar. Are there mineral supplements that could help?

▼
TIP:

Many minerals, including chromium, magnesium, selenium, and zinc, have been promoted by popular magazines and supplement companies as effective tools in controlling blood glucose. But there is currently no scientific evidence for these claims, so it is hard to recommend taking supplements. If you eat healthy foods, including lots of fresh fruits, vegetables, and grains, you should get all the minerals you need to stay healthy. From what we know now, taking supplements probably won't make you any healthier. Nor will it make your blood glucose any lower.

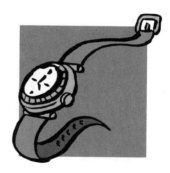

I'm so tired of checking my blood glucose. Will there ever be a way to check without sticking myself?

▼
TIP:

Several companies are working on so-called *non-invasive* blood glucose monitoring alternatives that work to get accurate blood glucose readings without the dreaded "poke."

The newest devices, however, are really only a step toward truly non-invasive monitoring. One looks like a wristwatch and you wear it on your wrist, just like a watch. You have to check your glucose the old fashioned way once a day to set the watch, which then gives glucose readings three times each hour.

Another company has a monitor about the size of a pager that gets readings through a sensor inserted under your skin. The monitor records glucose levels every 15 minutes. Since the device is new, the company has only limited approval. Your doctor has to give you the monitors, and they can only be used for a few days. The device stores all your glucose readings during that time, but you can't see them until you visit your doctor at the end of your monitoring period. If further testing is positive, this may change.

Hopefully, like the process of sterilizing and sharpening syringes before an injection, "sticking" yourself will soon fade into history, existing only as a memory of the diabetes therapy of old.

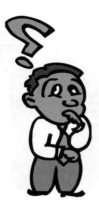

*W*ith *dozens of blood glucose monitors on the market, how do I choose the one that's right for me?*

TIP:

Picking the right monitor is a little like choosing a car—you have to think of the features that matter most to you. And there are lots of features to choose from. Are you looking for the fastest monitor? There are some that complete the check in 5 seconds. Other monitors have larger screens that are easier to see if your vision is not good. Some use strips that are easier to handle if you have arthritis or nerve damage. Looking to get organized? There are monitors that have lots of data management capabilities, which can help you track your results more precisely and communicate these results to your health care provider. There are monitors that use very small drops of blood and others that let you test on your hand, arm, or leg, as well as your finger.

So you see, there are lots of options. To choose the monitor that's best for you, talk to your health care provider. Or better yet, talk to a diabetes educator; he or she will probably be up to date on all the latest models and have some available for you to see.

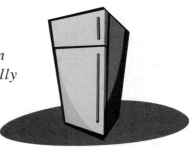

It is really hard to keep my insulin refrigerated all the time, especially when I travel. Do I always have to do this?

▼
TIP:

No. Your insulin should be fine for about 1 month as long as it does not freeze or get really hot—about 85° F. So as long as it is less than a month old, you only need to protect it from extreme temperatures. If you leave your insulin in a car on a hot summer day, keep it in a cooler—just make sure the insulin doesn't touch the ice, or it might freeze. You also need to be careful your insulin doesn't freeze in the winter. Keep it some place safe. And do the same when you fly. Always keep your insulin with you; never put it in the luggage you check. Your luggage could get lost, and even if it arrives safely, your insulin could be frozen or exposed to extreme heat.

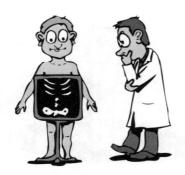

*D*o I really need to have an A1C check at the doctor's office if I check my blood glucose regularly at home?

▼

TIP:

The A1C check (also known as an HbA1c check) tells you your glucose control over a period of about 3 months. The glucose check you do at home tells you your level at that moment; the A1C tells you what your mean blood glucose has been over the last 90 days or so. The A1C check is a great tool because it gives a very clear, longer-term picture of your glucose control. That helps fill out the picture you get from your own glucose monitoring. For example, if your A1C level is 9%, your blood glucose averaged 210 mg/dl over the past 3 months. Unfortunately, this is about the average A1C of people with diabetes in the United States.

People who don't have diabetes have A1C levels somewhere under 6% (an average blood sugar of 90 mg/dl). As you can see, there is a big difference between normal blood glucose levels and the levels most people with diabetes have. The Diabetes Control and Complications Trial (DCCT) showed that lowering your A1C by just 0.5%, can make a big difference in your diabetes management. Getting your blood glucose levels closer to normal is hard work, but every little bit you lower them helps. The A1C test lets you see where you stand. You can use that information to increase your chances for a longer, healthier life.

I'm really confused about what my blood glucose level should be.

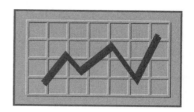

▼
TIP:

The simple answer is, as close to normal as possible. The ADA recommends specific glucose goals for people with diabetes. They say you should aim for glucose levels that are 80–120 mg/dl before meals, for levels less than 160 mg/dl 2 hours after meals, and for levels that are 100–140 mg/dl before bed. As for A1C, they suggest you aim for a level of near or under 7%—an average glucose of about 150 mg/dl. The ADA has also set higher "take action" levels for each of these measures. For example, the "take action" level for A1C is 8% (an average glucose level of 180 mg/dl).

If your current glucose levels are higher than the ADA goals, or even if they're higher than the take action levels, don't lose heart. At last half of all people with diabetes in this country have A1C levels higher than the ADA "take action" level. The most important message is this: every little bit helps. If you lower your glucose and keep it lower, you lower your risk of diabetes complications. That's as true for people who have A1C levels of 11% as it is for those whose levels are much lower.

Chapter 5
MANAGING HIGH AND
LOW BLOOD GLUCOSE

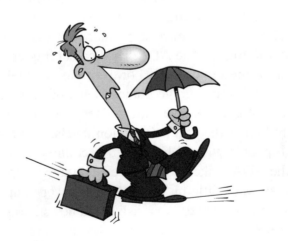

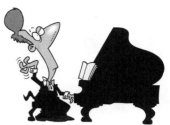

*H*ow can I treat a low blood
glucose when I am at the theater
or a concert without making lots of
noise unwrapping candy?

▼
TIP:

Put jellybeans (or some other "soft" candy) into a plastic sand-
wich bag. The plastic bag makes no noise when opened, and the
candy won't make any noise when you chew it. Make sure you
know how many candies you need to treat a typical low and make
up a bunch of single-use "bean bags." That way you will have a
ready source of tasty, portion-controlled carbohydrate whenever you
need it. Keep one in your briefcase, car, bedside stand, and anywhere else it might come in handy.

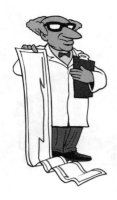

*H*ow can I resist taking too much insulin
to treat a high blood glucose?

▼
TIP:

Instead of treating a high blood glucose in one big swoop, take it
down in small steps. Trying to get your blood glucose down when
it is high is a good thing. But overdoing it can push your level too
low, and that isn't a good thing. So you have to think before treating—what has worked in the past and what hasn't? It would be
great if you could go from a high glucose level to a normal one in
one big jump, with a nice, soft landing. But it usually doesn't work
that way; sometimes the landing is hard. Too often you end up low,
and that hurts. To avoid that, get your blood glucose back where you
want it in a couple of easier steps, instead of one giant, painful step.
Take a little less insulin than is tempting, and then check your glucose level when the insulin should be working to see the results and
make any adjustments. This approach should make it possible to get
your blood glucose down while lowering the risk of going too low.

Why shouldn't I eat chocolate to treat a low?

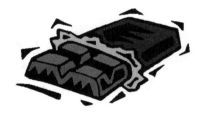

▼
TIP:

Many people are tempted to eat chocolate to treat a low, because they love chocolate and they feel they are making good of a bad situation. To some degree they are, but this approach has a downside. Chocolate contains a lot of fat, which is part of the reason it tastes so good. Unfortunately, your body absorbs foods that contain fat more slowly, so something sugary and fat-free will probably raise your glucose faster than chocolate. So, though it might be tempting to reach for the chocolates when you are low, other things will probably get you back to normal quicker. That doesn't mean you shouldn't enjoy chocolate. Just be aware of its limits as a treatment for low blood glucose.

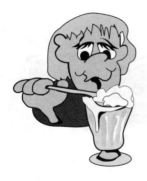

*H*ow can I avoid overeating when I am low?

It's easy to overeat when you are low, because a low blood glucose makes it very hard to think clearly. Everything you know about food and how much it takes to bring your glucose up without going too high goes out the window. Instead, you respond to something that is very clear: your body's cry of "feed me!" By the time you're thinking clearly again, you have usually eaten way too much.

A few things can help make it easier to resist temptation:

- First, have unit-size low glucose treatment "kits" available. These can be anything that works for you, from a small box of raisins to a can of regular soda to a few jelly beans.
- Second, when you are low, get one of your kits and take it somewhere away from other sources of food.
- Third, eat what is in your kit and tell yourself something simple that helps you wait 15 minutes before taking any further action (unless, of course, you feel *worse*). An example: "I really want more but this is probably enough." Keep your phrase simple or you won't be able to keep it in mind when you are low.

I *had a really bad low blood sugar*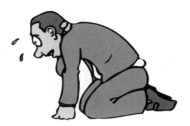
and my doctor told me I needed
to get glucagon. What is glucagon?

▼
TIP:

G lucagon is an emergency treatment that is prescribed by your
doctor for severe low blood glucose. It is injected when your
reaction is so severe you can't treat yourself with food or drink,
whether it's from an inability to swallow, confusion, or even uncon-
sciousness. Since you won't be in any condition to give yourself
glucagon when you need it, someone else should know when to give
it and how to mix and inject the glucagon shot. It will usually raise
your blood glucose in about 10–15 minutes.

Having glucagon (and someone who knows how to use it!)
readily available can mean the difference between a scary few
minutes and a much longer ordeal with 911 calls and trips to the
emergency room. Keep in mind that glucagon raises your blood
glucose by drawing on the glucose reserves in your liver, so you
should eat something as soon as you can to replace those reserves.
Unfortunately, some people feel sick to their stomach after taking
glucagon, so eat lightly.

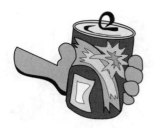

What is the best treatment for low blood glucose?

There are lots of choices. The ADA recommends you treat a low glucose level (less than 70 mg/dl) by eating or drinking something that contains 15 grams of sugar, preferably in a form that is absorbed quickly. Good choices include hard candy, jelly beans, fruit, fruit juice, regular soda, honey, table sugar, and glucose tablets or gel. Look up your favorite low blood glucose treatment foods to see how much of each equals 15 grams.

Check your glucose level 15 minutes after eating and treat again if you are still low. Try to avoid overtreating lows, and don't eat pure chocolate to treat lows because it contains lots of fat and relatively little sugar, so it takes longer to raise your blood glucose.

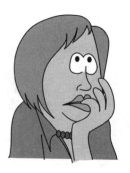

I *have to take a lot more insulin just before I get my period. Is that normal?*

▼

TIP:

Many women find they need more insulin in the days just before they start to menstruate, and that their insulin needs go back to normal when their periods begin. This isn't surprising, since estrogen levels increase just before a woman's period begins, and estrogen raises insulin needs. Everyone is different—your menstrual cycle might have a tremendous effect on your glucose levels or it might have none at all. Younger women tend to have this menstrual fluctuation most dramatically. If your blood sugars go up before your period, try to figure out when it starts to happen and try to pin down the amount of additional insulin you'll need until your period begins.

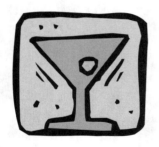

I got really low once when my friends and I were drinking, and they thought I was drunk. How can they tell the difference in the future?

TIP:

First of all, drinking too much is never a good idea. Your friends should not be responsible for your low blood sugar or your diabetes. The signs of going low and being drunk are very similar, and it will be hard for them to tell which is at work, especially if they've been drinking too. If you take insulin, the problem can be even worse, because drinking too much can lower glucose levels even more.

Do all you can to avoid going low when you are drinking. Eat a little something extra. Take a little less insulin. Check your blood glucose when you can. Once again, your friends should not be responsible for you, but some friends will want to know how to help. He or she must be sober and must be able to recognize changes in your behavior that indicate you might be low. Your friend should also know how to check your blood glucose level and know what to do if you are low or it's impossible to check your glucose. The easiest remedy in this situation is 4–6 ounces (about half of a glass) of regular (not diet) soft drink. This will be helpful if you're low and harmless if you've just had a little too much to drink.

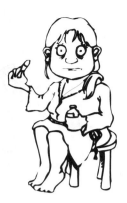

*H*igh *blood glucose levels after meals really upset me. Is there anything I can do to keep them down?*

▼
TIP:

To avoid high glucose after a meal, you need information. Check your levels before eating and again 2 hours later. Do this for each meal a couple of times. If you take rapid acting insulin with your meals, you can use your after-meal glucose levels to figure out how much more insulin you need to take before you eat. Be sure to talk with your health care provider before making changes in your plan—adding insulin can increase your risk of going too low. Some diabetes pills are especially effective for helping control after-meal glucose levels (for example, repaglinide [Prandin] and nateglinide [Starlix]). Talk to your health care provider about these pills if you are not already taking them. Taking a walk after eating can help, too. So can eating smaller, more frequent meals or eating meals with less carbohydrate, since carbohydrates contribute most to after-meal high glucose levels.

The fact you check your levels and know your after-meal blood glucose level is a good thing. Most people don't know because they rarely check. And unfortunately, most people have higher glucose levels after meals than they do before meals. Researchers say that after-meal glucose levels contribute to as much as one-third of A1C levels, the standard measure of long-term control.

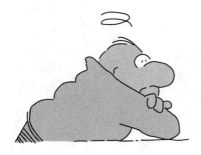

I strive for tight control, and I'm very scared of getting complications. How can I keep from getting really upset every time I get a high blood glucose?

▼
TIP:

Try not to worry. An occasional spike in your blood glucose is not likely to cause any harm. The problems come when your blood glucose stays high for long periods of time—days, weeks, and months. The best predictor of your chances for a long life, free of complications such as heart disease and stroke, is your average blood glucose level over a period of months (along with your blood pressure and lipid levels), not the number of blood sugar spikes. The A1C test gives the best estimate of your long-term control and risk of diabetes complications. Many studies have shown that whether you have type 1 diabetes or type 2, the lower your A1C, the lower your risk of developing complications. So your A1C level is the number to focus on, not a particular glucose reading. Focusing on individual blood sugar readings is misleading, and if you concentrate on the high ones it is likely to sap your motivation and energy. You need a realistic perspective to support the hard work required to manage your diabetes, and that perspective should be broader than your most recent glucose reading.

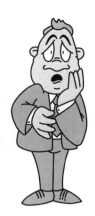

I was shocked at how high my last A1C was. How could it be high when my morning blood glucose checks are always close to normal?

▼
TIP:

Your blood glucose levels can change quite a bit during the day, which means checking at a single time each day can give a very misleading picture of your overall control. The glucose checks you do at home are like photographs; they capture what is going on the moment they are done. On the other hand, an A1C reading is like a 3-month-long videotape; it captures everything that goes on during that period. As you can imagine, the videotape contains much more information about those 3 months than a daily photograph would.

For example, if someone took a single photograph of you each day at 3:00 A.M. for 3 months and then used the photographs to see what you did for those 3 months, it would look like you had been sleeping the whole time. In the same way, if your blood glucose tends to be lowest in the morning, those readings won't give an accurate picture of your overall control. Talk to your health care provider about checking at other times of the day to see when you are high, and what you can do to get your overall control in line with your good morning levels.

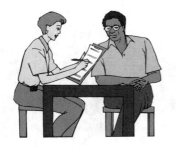

*W*hat should my A1C be to avoid complications?

There is no magic A1C number that guarantees you will not develop complications. However, the lower your A1C level, the less likely you are to get diabetes complications. It now seems that even slightly elevated A1C levels carry some increased risk for complications like heart disease and stroke. Unfortunately, very few people can get their A1C levels as low as they are in people who don't have diabetes; we don't have the tools to achieve this goal, and the amount of work and the increased risk of low blood glucose make it impossible for most people to manage. So all people with diabetes carry some increased risk of developing complications. Trying to be realistic, the American Diabetes Association says people with diabetes should aim for A1C levels of 7% or less. That's the equivalent of a 150 mg/dl average blood glucose. The ADA suggests that you take action and talk with your health care provider about changes in your treatment if your A1C is higher than 8% (the equivalent of a 180 mg/dl average blood glucose). The most important thing to keep in mind is this: Any improvement in your A1C reduces your risk of getting diabetes complications. A small improvement reduces your risk a little, and a big improvement reduces your risk a lot. But every improvement reduces your risk.

Chapter 6
UNDERSTANDING AND
AVOIDING COMPLICATIONS

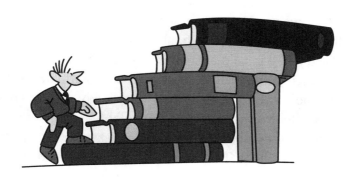

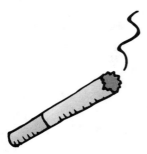

I don't think I can quit smoking. How important is it for me to stop?

▼

TIP:

Very. Smoking is unhealthy for anyone, but smoking and diabetes is a truly deadly combination. Even if you didn't smoke, your risk of getting heart disease or having a stroke increases 2–4 times just because you have diabetes. Diabetes can cause blocked arteries, which leads to heart attacks and strokes. Smoking makes this even worse, and the risk of serious heart problems when you have diabetes *and* smoke is about 10 times greater than for someone who doesn't have diabetes or smoke.

You can't change the fact you have diabetes, but hard as it is, you can stop smoking. If you decide you are ready to stop smoking, there are many effective help programs available. Contact the American Lung Association in your area, or ask your physician or diabetes educator for help. They may refer you to a good stop-smoking program in your area. Nicotine patches and nicotine gum are also available from the drugstore, and they can help you deal with your nicotine addiction while you stop smoking.

It's hard enough trying to control my blood sugars. Do I have to control my blood pressure and lipid levels as well?

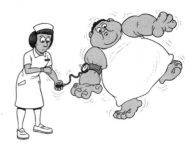

▼

TIP:

Controlling your blood pressure and lipid (cholesterol) levels is as important as controlling your blood sugar, if not even more important. Heart attacks and stroke are the major causes of death among people with diabetes, and your risk of developing these complications is 2–4 times greater than for someone without diabetes. High blood pressure and abnormal lipids are major risk factors for these complications.

In addition to reducing stress, increasing activity, and eating heart healthy meals, there are excellent medications available to help you control blood pressure and lipids. The recommended levels for people with diabetes are lower than the levels for people the same age who don't have diabetes, due to the fact that people with diabetes are at a higher risk. Current goals for people with diabetes are:

- Blood pressure <130/80
- LDL cholesterol (the bad one) <100
- HDL cholesterol (the good cholesterol) >45.

Talk to your health care provider about your levels and anything you can do to improve them.

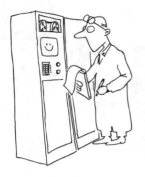

*I*s the trouble I'm having with my erections related to my diabetes?

TIP:

Quite possibly, but maybe not. Millions of men who don't have diabetes still have trouble getting and keeping an erection. The causes may be physical or psychological or both. Still, problems with erections are more common in men with diabetes, and the causes are usually physical. Diabetes can affect the nerves and the blood vessels that control erections. Ask you doctor to help you identify what could be causing your erection problems. In addition to blood vessel and nerve damage, your doctor might talk to you about the possibility that depression or drinking too much alcohol could be contributing to your problems. They might even be a side effect of a medication you're taking.

There are many treatments available, such as improving blood glucose control, taking medications such as Viagra that make it easier to get and keep an erection, or using devices designed to do the same thing. Devices include simple elastic rings that prevent blood from flowing back out of the penis (and thereby prevent losing the erection) to penile implants that require surgery.

Ask your primary care provider for a referral to a physician who specializes in diagnosing and treating erection problems. Usually this will be a urologist.

*C*an diabetes affect a woman's sexuality?

▼
TIP:

Diabetes can affect a woman's sexual experience in a variety of ways. Some women have problems with vaginal dryness, and that can make intercourse uncomfortable. Having diabetes also increases your risk for infections, including vaginal infections. Nerve damage can dramatically reduce sensation and pleasure. Limited mobility, feeling unattractive because of weight, and feeling tired because of high glucose levels all contribute further to the challenges many women with diabetes face when it comes to their sexuality.

Fortunately, there are ways to deal with these challenges, though none is perfect and they all take work. Be sure to talk with your health care provider about your options. Vaginal lubricants can relieve dryness. Controlling your blood sugar and using a medication can help control yeast infections. Learning the touch you can feel and enjoy is very important if you have nerve damage. Building strength through exercise, and finding comfortable positions can help if you have limited mobility. Focusing on what makes you attractive—you know there are things that do—is the last and most important element of a plan for a more enjoyable sex life.

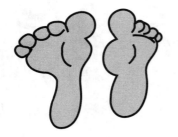

I've had a lot of trouble with my feet. They used to hurt and burn, but now I hardly feel them at all. Are things getting better?

▼ TIP:

Probably not. It sounds as if you have neuropathy, or nerve damage, which is common in people who have had diabetes for many years. As nerve damage gets worse, people often notice the very symptoms you describe: lots of burning and pain at first, but then much less as time goes on. Many times people say they no longer feel their feet at all. While pain can be awful, when you lose feeling in your feet you also lose an important warning sign. Pain has a purpose. If your foot hurts when you step on a tack, for instance, you will quickly remove the tack and treat the wound. But when you don't feel pain you lose the protection it provides. You don't feel anything when you step on the tack, so unless you frequently check your feet, it can take a long time for you to realize you're in trouble and to take action. That delay can lead to infections, and infections can be especially hard to clear up when you have diabetes. So going from painful feet to feet you can't feel is not a good thing. Your feet hurt less, but that means you need to find other ways to protect them.

I have one diabetes complication and feel like lots more will follow. Does having one complication mean I will get others?

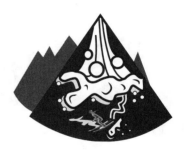

▼
TIP:

Not necessarily. It is true that higher blood glucose levels make all complications more likely, so if high glucose levels have led to one complication, they may very well lead to others. But you can use this correlation to your advantage. If your blood glucose levels go down, you lower your chances of getting another complication. Not only that, but getting your glucose levels down is one of the best ways to keep the complication you already have from getting worse.

Doing your best to stay healthy is hard because it takes so much time and effort. Keeping in mind why you try so hard can help maintain your motivation. Some people say that getting a complication made them see their lives with diabetes differently; the complication was both a blow and a wake-up call. It hurts and it makes them take a hard look at how they were managing their diabetes. Talk to your health care provider about things you can do to increase your chances of living the rest of your life with no more complications.

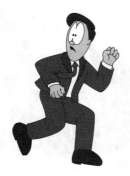

How can I stop worrying so much about high blood sugars? My fears make me keep my level too low much of the time.

▼

TIP:

Keeping your blood glucose levels close to normal is a good thing. It helps you feel better day-to-day, and it cuts your risk for diabetes complications. Unfortunately, it sounds as if you push so hard for the lowest possible glucose levels that it actually makes you feel worse. Being low a lot is a burden. It's embarrassing and it can be dangerous. People who are often low also tend to worry about it almost constantly. So they worry about highs and they worry about lows.

It's hard not to worry about your blood glucose levels, but sometimes it helps to look at the facts. First, what is your A1C level? If it is under 8%, your control is pretty good. If it is under 7%, it is very good. There is much room for improvement if your A1C level is higher than 8%. That would mean you are having lots of highs along with the lows. Talk to your health care provider about changes in your treatment plan that could help keep your glucose levels closer to normal throughout the day and cut down on your worrying.

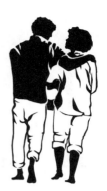

I *think diabetes caused my wife's heart attack. Is there anything we can do to help avoid another one?*

▼

TIP:

Having diabetes certainly made your wife's heart attack more likely. Heart disease is the leading cause of death in people with diabetes. There are things your wife—and you—can do to help protect her from another heart attack. She can try to live a healthier life by staying active, cutting the amount of fat she eats, controlling her weight, and taking medication (if prescribed) to help with other risk factors like her blood pressure and cholesterol levels. If your wife smokes, stopping is the most important thing she could do to keep her heart healthy.

Making these changes is hard, and that is where you come in. Give your wife the support she needs. Ask what you can do to help, whether it is preparing a healthy, tasty dinner or joining her for a walk after you have enjoyed your meal. You could also help your wife find useful diabetes resources, such as education classes, a good dietitian, or Internet websites. Getting involved in a positive way like this can do you both good.

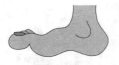

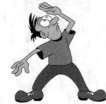

*H*ow *can I check my feet every night like I am supposed to when my eyesight is so bad?*

▼

TIP:

U nfortunately, you are not alone. As important as it is to check your feet every day, especially if you have any loss of feeling, many people have trouble checking themselves because of back, vision, or other problems. You may be able to rig up a system that lets you see your feet. Shining a flashlight on your feet or placing a lamp on the floor right by your feet while you check them could help. If you have trouble seeing the bottom of your feet, place a mirror on the floor and hold your foot over it.

If you still aren't able to check your feet yourself, ask family members or friends to help. It's hard to ask for help, but if there are people in your life who love you and have the time, it's worth asking. They might even appreciate the chance to do it. Talk to your health care provider about other ways to help your feet last a lifetime.

*W*ill a pill solve my sexual problems?

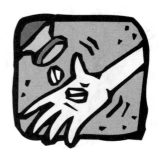

▼
TIP:

It could help. There is a pill called Viagra that men take to help them maintain erections. Studies show the pill is safe, and it seems to help many men who have diabetes. In one study, men taking Viagra said they had good erections about half the time they tried intercourse, while men taking a placebo medication said they had good erections only about 10% of the time.

Some people who use Viagra have side effects, especially headaches, flushing, and indigestion. People who take nitroglycerine for heart problems or any other nitrate medication should not take Viagra because their blood pressure could fall dangerously low. Researchers are still studying the effects of Viagra, including any benefits it might provide for women.

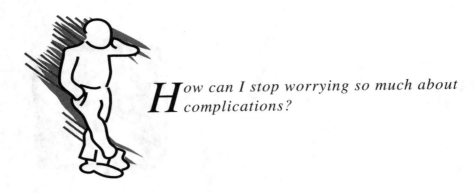

How can I stop worrying so much about complications?

▼
TIP:

First, do everything you can to prevent them. Keeping your blood glucose close to normal makes complications less likely, and that might help you worry less. Talk to your health care providers on a regular basis. They can help you take better care of yourself and check to see if you have any signs of complications, so any problems can be treated as quickly as possible. Knowing you have good care and good control can put a lot of fears to rest.

Share your feelings with family or friends who might be able to offer support. Consider joining a diabetes support group. There you will see that your feelings are not that unusual (and probably pick up some new tips for improving your glucose control). It can also help to connect with the sources of confidence and peace of mind that mean the most to you. Religious faith can be a tremendous source of strength and serenity, and so can the loving support of family and friends or the confidence you feel in yourself when you know you are taking good care of yourself.

Finally, consider this homily: "Worry never robs tomorrow of its sorrow; it only saps today of its strength."

*I*s it true that I have to give up alcohol?

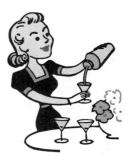

No. If your blood glucose control is good, having an occasional drink with meals should do no harm. The dietary guidelines published by the U.S. government say drinking moderately is okay as long as you don't drink and drive. Moderate drinking means one drink a day for women and two for men. One drink is 12 ounces of regular beer, 5 ounces of wine, or 1-1/2 ounces of 80-proof distilled spirits. These guidelines work for most people who have diabetes.

Having diabetes means you should also take special precautions when it comes to drinking. First, you need to fit the calories you are drinking into your meal plan to avoid going too high. That's important because alcohol contains almost as many calories per gram as fat does. Substitute alcohol calories for fat calories, with one drink equal to about 90 calories. Second, alcohol can cause very low blood glucose if you drink and don't eat anything. If you take insulin or pills that help your body make more insulin (sulfonylureas or meglitinides), it is safest to drink alcohol only with meals.

So it is okay to drink, but as with so many other things, it takes extra effort to do it safely when you have diabetes.

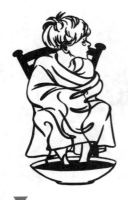

I'm worried about this sore on my foot that the doctor called a foot ulcer. What is a foot ulcer?

An ulcer is an open sore. People with diabetes are more likely to get foot ulcers for three reasons. First, many people with diabetes have lost some feeling in their feet because of nerve damage, so they might not notice tiny cuts or cracks in the skin that could lead to serious problems. Second, many people with diabetes also have circulation problems, so it is hard to get oxygen, white blood cells, and antibiotics to the wound to help it heal. That's why many people with diabetes find that any wound, even the smallest one, can take a really long time to heal. In fact, without an adequate blood supply, foot ulcers may never heal. Finally, high blood glucose levels also hinder healing.

Foot ulcers can appear any place on your feet, though most often they are on the bottom or side of your big toe and on the ball of the foot. Prevention is essential. Pamper your feet. Keep them clean, dry, and protected from injury. Watch them like a hawk. If you see any sign of an open cut or sore, no matter how small, contact your health care provider immediately. You might also ask for a referral to a podiatrist, someone who specializes in treating foot problems.

*H*ow can I have diabetes complications when I don't feel bad?

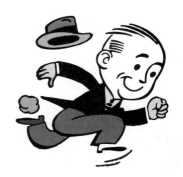

▼

TIP:

Unfortunately, you can feel fine without really being fine. For example, people with diabetes often have nerve damage, so they don't feel things that indicate serious problems. Like heart problems, for example. People who have diabetes are more likely to suffer so-called silent heart attacks, serious heart damage they never even feel. Serious foot problems are also more common in people who have diabetes, in part for the same reason—nerve damage caused by the disease. Small foot injuries are often overlooked because the person doesn't feel bad. In fact, the person might not feel anything at all, even with a very serious foot ulcer.

So you can have complications and not feel bad. Just as important, you can have a very high risk of developing complications without feeling bad. Many people walk around for years with dangerously high glucose levels, and say they do not feel bad. So what you can't feel can hurt you. That is why it is so important to have regular checkups with your health care provider and verify that everything you can't feel is okay. That will help protect you from feeling bad for years to come.

Chapter 7
GETTING THE BEST
HEALTH CARE

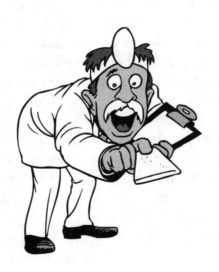

Should I be seeing any specialists for my diabetes?

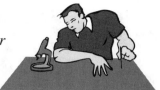

This is a terrific question with no clear-cut answers. Many primary care practitioners, or generalists, know a lot about diabetes and try to keep up to date. You are reading this book, so you are learning a lot about diabetes. If you believe your practitioner is not as up to date as you or is not giving you the care or answers you desire, you should look for another practitioner or request a referral to a specialist. Endocrinologists specialize in treating diseases of the endocrine system, including diabetes. However, not all endocrinologists specialize in diabetes, so try to find one who does.

No matter what, you should see an eye care specialist. If you are having problems with your feet you should see a podiatrist. You should also see specialists if you have problems with your heart, or have kidney or nerve damage. Diabetes educators can help you build your self-care skills, and mental health professionals can help you cope with the stresses of life with diabetes. Talk with your health care provider to be sure you have all the right players on your diabetes care team, and to decide how often you should see each of them.

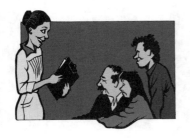

I just got diabetes and I am confused about what I need to do. Should I see a diabetes educator?

▼
TIP:

Yes. A diabetes educator can help you get off to a good start living with diabetes. Among other things, a diabetes educator can help you learn:

- How to check your blood glucose
- How and when to take insulin or diabetes pills (if this applies to you)
- How to recognize when your glucose is too high or low and what to do about it
- How to eat healthier and be more active
- How to quit smoking (if you are a smoker)

Diabetes educators are a great source of continuing support and helpful information and should be key members of your diabetes treatment team in the future, as well.

Many insurance plans, including Medicare, will pay for diabetes education. The ADA has a list of education programs they formally recognize on their website (*www.diabetes.org*). Or call 1-800-DIABETES for information. You can also contact the American Association of Diabetes Educators (AADE) at 1-800-TEAM-UP-4 or *www.aadenet.org* to get the names of diabetes educators in your area. Your local hospital may also offer diabetes education programs or have a diabetes educator on staff.

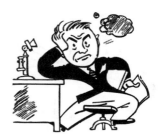

I *can't find time during my doctor appointments to get my questions answered. What should I do?*

▼
TIP:

■ Write down the issues you want to discuss before your visit. Your health care provider has limited time, so stay simple and focus on the things that matter most. You might see if the person checking you in can place a copy of the list in your chart for the provider to see. Tell your provider right away that you have questions so there is time to get answers.

■ Make sure your questions are complete and reflect your true concerns. A complete question might be, "Which protein source is lowest in fat?" or "How can I avoid being so worried about my heart?"

■ Your physician may respond to faxes, though some prefer not to communicate this way. If your provider does respond to faxes (or phone calls), limit the exchange to 1 or 2 short, simple questions. E-mail may also be a possibility.

■ Health care providers are experts in the medical management of diabetes; you are the expert in your life with diabetes. As they share their knowledge about diabetes with you, share with them your knowledge about your life and let them know what makes diabetes management more difficult. This is the best way to solve problems and reach your diabetes goals.

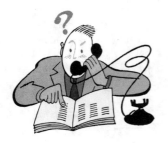

I just moved to a new city. How do I find a good diabetes doctor?

▼
TIP:

You could ask your previous doctor for a referral, contact a local hospital in your new city, or get in touch with the American Diabetes Association (1-800-DIABETES). You could also find a diabetes educator in your new city and ask him or her. Call the American Association of Diabetes Educators' referral line, 1-800-TEAM-UP-4 (or go to the AADE web site, *www.aadenet.org*). Attending a diabetes support group (most local hospitals have them) and asking people about their doctors is also an option.

When you consider a new doctor, keep in mind the things that matter most to you. Important factors include:

- Your insurance coverage
- How much the doctor seems to know about diabetes
- The doctor's personal style
- The availability of a diabetes treatment team (nurse, dietitian, and others)
- How easy it is to get to the office

A good diabetes doctor can be a tremendous resource, so do all you can to choose yours wisely.

I don't like the way my
diabetes is being treated.
What can I do about it?

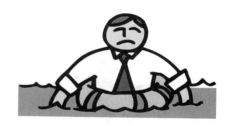

▼
TIP:

First, talk to your health care provider. Explain to him or her that you are not happy with your current treatment, explain why you are not happy, and ask what you can do to get your treatment more to your liking. Another option is to try "smart experiments," where you change elements of your diabetes treatment to get the most benefits and the least problems. One example would be switching your exercise to after dinner to see if it helps control evening blood sugars. The rules for smart experiments are:

- Always discuss them first with your health care provider. He or she can help you refine your plan and point out any possible dangers.
- Know the diabetes basics before you start. For example, how your diabetes medications affect your glucose levels, how to measure your blood glucose, and how to recognize symptoms of low and high glucose.
- Start with one or two changes. Monitor frequently to check the results of your experiment.
- Don't make big changes. Make smaller ones, especially at first.
- Keep good records of what you are doing—changes in medication dose and timing, when you eat, exercise, and so on. This makes it easier to figure out what works best for you.

If you don't like how your diabetes is being treated, smart experiments could help.

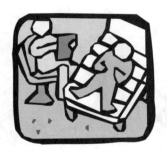

*S*hould I see a mental health
professional for my diabetes?

▼
TIP:

It could be a good idea. Many people who have diabetes feel
"stressed-out" by the daily demands of their disease. Feeling overwhelmed is terrible, and it can trigger a negative spiral—if you feel
overwhelmed, you probably can't find the energy to actively care for
your diabetes, so your glucose control suffers. That means you feel
worse physically and worry a lot about the long-term damage
caused by those high glucose levels. And that creates even more
stress.

So, doing anything you can to cut stress is very good. Doing
things you enjoy and getting support from family and friends can
help, and so can talking to a good counselor. If you have more serious emotional problems, like depression, the need for professional
help is even greater. Working with a mental health professional who
knows something about diabetes could help you feel better and get
you back on track with your diabetes care. Unfortunately, there aren't
many mental health professionals who specialize in working with
people who have diabetes. To see if there are any in your area, ask
you health care provider, contact your local hospital, call the ADA at
1-800-DIABETES, or call the AADE at 1-800-TEAM-UP-4.

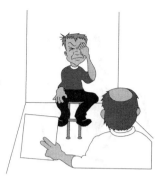

I'm having vision problems. Are there any specialists I should see?

▼

TIP:

Absolutely. Eye problems are a common complication of diabetes and an ophthalmologist (a doctor who specializes in eye care) can help preserve your sight. An ophthalmologist can tell if your eyes have been affected by diabetes. If so, an eye doctor can treat your eyes with laser therapy to protect your vision. Because it protects so many people from blindness, this treatment is one of the great advances in diabetes care over the past 30 years. Laser therapy works best if it is performed at the first sign of eye problems, which is why regular visits to the eye doctor are so important.

The ADA recommends you have a complete eye exam with an eye doctor every year if you were diagnosed with diabetes after you were 30 years old, or if you are younger and have had diabetes at least 5 years. Try to find an eye doctor who has experience treating people with diabetes. Ask your health care provider for a referral.

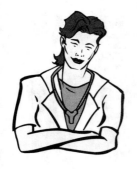

My mother had serious foot problems with her diabetes and I am afraid the same thing could happen to me. Should I see a foot doctor?

▼
TIP:

Yes. Foot care is very important when you have diabetes, and seeing a podiatrist (foot doctor) will help you keep your feet healthy. Because you have diabetes, you are more likely to have nerve damage (which means you can hurt your feet without feeling it) and circulation problems (which means any injuries to your feet take a really long time to heal). To help, a podiatrist can:

- Show you how to care for your feet at home
- Help you with routine foot care, which can prevent more serious problems
- Treat corns, calluses, and small sores
- Help you keep your toenails safely trimmed
- Design supports to protect your foot from pressures that create sores
- Show you how to buy shoes that fit properly
- Perform foot surgery, to help save feet from even more serious harm

Ask your health care provider for a referral to a podiatrist if you have any questions or concerns about your feet. Local hospitals or the local ADA office can also help you find a podiatrist.

I'm worried my health insurance
isn't good enough. What should be
covered by my insurance plan?

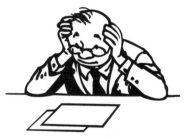

▼

TIP:

The ADA says your health care coverage should include the
following:

- Regular health care visits (yearly eye exams, as well as 4 visits a
  year with your regular doctor if you have type 1 diabetes, and
  2 times a year if you have type 2 diabetes)
- Lab tests (including tests of A1C, blood pressure, and blood fat
  levels, as well as tests to monitor any complications)
- All the diabetes medications and supplies you need for good care
  (including blood monitors and strips)
- Diabetes education provided by trained educators. After all, you
  provide most of your own diabetes care, and you need to know
  how to do it.

Unfortunately, many people with diabetes do not have this kind
of coverage. Insurance companies are hesitant to cover people with
conditions like diabetes because they can be costly to treat. Things
are beginning to shift, and benefits are improving under both private
and government health insurance plans. However, you might find
that your coverage is still not good. If you are not getting what the
ADA recommends, you are not getting what you deserve. Talk to
your health care provider or contact the ADA for help getting the
coverage you need.

Chapter 8
GETTING THE SUPPORT
AND INFORMATION
YOU NEED

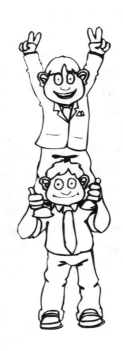

*H*ow can I get my family to be more supportive when it comes to my diabetes?

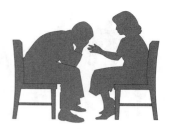

▼
TIP:

Many people who have diabetes are looking for more and better support from their families. Some feel their families don't take their diabetes seriously enough, don't understand the challenges of diabetes management, or don't accommodate their diabetes needs. Some feel their families even tempt them to take worse care of themselves. Other people feel their families go to the opposite extreme, forming a "diabetes police" that tries to control everything they do.

You need your family's positive support to live well with diabetes, but each person's need for this support is different. To help get the support *you* need, answer these three questions:

- What does my family do that makes my life with diabetes easier?
- What does my family do that makes my life with diabetes harder?
- What could my family (realistically) do differently to help me manage my diabetes?

Once you have answered these questions, talk with your family. Let them know how much you appreciate the help they are already providing, try to understand their feelings, and work to get more support one step at a time.

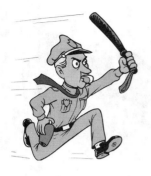

My husband has become the "diabetes police" and he's on me about everything I do and don't do. How can I get him to stop trying to control my diabetes?

TIP:

Keep in mind that your husband probably does this because he loves you and is worried that something bad will happen if he doesn't stay on your case. Unfortunately, this "diabetes police" approach does not work for either of you. You feel harassed, your husband feels frustrated and helpless—something has to change.

First, try to identify anything your husband does that actually helps you manage your diabetes. He seems to be looking for ways to help. Getting him to do more of the things you appreciate might shift the way you are relating to each other about diabetes management.

Once you know what you want from your husband, talk to him about it. Let him know that you appreciate his love and concern for you, but that his "policing" isn't helping. Be as specific as you can about what you want and need. Ask him to talk about how he *feels* ("I get really upset when I see you go for that second helping of dessert") instead of what you *do* ("How could you eat that when you know what it will do to your glucose?"). Talking about feelings and what your husband is already doing to help are good ways to get him to turn in his diabetes police badge for good.

*B*oth *my sister and I have diabetes, but she seems to take much better care of herself. How can I deal with this?*

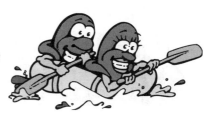

▼

TIP:

*M*any of us have siblings we envy for one reason or another—success, looks, or even the fact that they manage their diabetes better. While this can be a source of frustration, it can also be a source of motivation. Try to identify the things you admire about the way your sister manages her diabetes. Does your sister's approach help you see how you might manage your own diabetes better? If so, think about a step-by-step approach to working in some of those things into your own diabetes care.

It can also help to be clear about what you are already doing right when it comes to managing your diabetes. There are probably things you overlook when you are comparing yourself to your sister. There might even be some things you do better than she does.

Once you are feeling more confident about your own diabetes management, talk with your sister. You might be surprised to hear that she struggles with her diabetes more than you realize. Hopefully, you can both do better, and turn your shared situation from a source of sibling stress into a source of sibling strength.

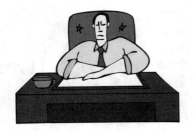

Should I tell a prospective employer I have diabetes?

TIP:

This is up to you. Job discrimination against people with diabetes has dropped over the years. According to current laws, you can only be denied a job if you can't perform the essential duties of the job even if the employer makes reasonable accommodations to help you (like providing breaks for you to check your glucose, have snacks, and go to the bathroom more frequently). Unfortunately, the new laws only cover people who work for companies that employ at least 15 people, and proving hiring discrimination is tough. Still, employers can get into big trouble if they reject a person who has diabetes and then hire a less qualified person.

Many employers will not ask about your health. In fact, it is illegal to do so unless they ask all prospective employees the same question. If your employer does ask, you don't have to tell them. However, you could lose some of your legal protections against job discrimination if you lie about having diabetes before you are hired.

Many people say it is best to tell because work is less stressful when they aren't trying to hide something as important as diabetes. It is also easier to take better care of your diabetes at work when you can do it openly.

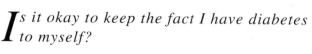 *s it okay to keep the fact I have diabetes to myself?*

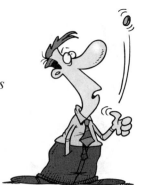

▼

TIP:

Once again, this is up to you. First, keep in mind that diabetes is pretty common now, so many people know a little about diabetes. Second, diabetes is not a disease to be ashamed of. It is not caused by improper behavior.

Most people are curious about something that they may have heard about, but don't really understand. They will naturally have questions. Humor can be a useful tool to help break the tension you may feel talking about your diabetes. For instance:

"I would have never known you had diabetes!"

"Well they stopped making us wear the scarlet Ds a long time ago!"

It may be uncomfortable, but it's a good idea to let people you spend lots of time with (like your co-workers) know you could go low (if this is a possibility), how you act when you are low, and how to help you treat the low if you can't do it yourself. If you pick the right people to tell, you will probably get some understanding right away, and possibly some needed help in case of an emergency later.

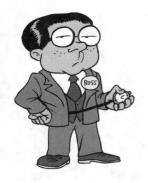

My boss gives me a hard time when I take a break to get a snack because my blood glucose is low. What can I do?

TIP:

Your boss's behavior is illegal. As long as you are able to get your work done, you should be allowed reasonable accommodations, including breaks for snacks, glucose checks, and more trips to the restroom. You should also be allowed to keep food and diabetes supplies nearby and be allowed to work a standard shift instead of a swing shift. If you're not getting these things, your boss is breaking the law.

Consider making your own accommodations (but none that compromise your health!) to make it easier for your employer to follow the law and meet your needs. If your boss refuses to cooperate, talk to the human resources department at your company. Provide the following to anyone you talk to:

■ Information about diabetes
■ What you do to manage your diabetes
■ Specific accommodations you require
■ The company's legal obligation to provide those accommodations under the law.

If all else fails, you might contact organizations dedicated to fighting job discrimination, such as the ADA, your union (if you belong to one), your state human rights commission, the Equal Employment Opportunity Commission, the U.S. Department of Labor, or your local employment office.

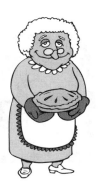

*W*hat should I say to a friend who tempts me with things I shouldn't eat, saying a little bit won't hurt me?

First, be sure your friend understands why you don't want to eat what he or she is offering. Be as specific as you can. Maybe you are afraid of a high glucose, or worried you would not be able to stop after eating a little bit. Or it could be that you simply don't want anything to eat. Whatever your reason, give it. That should stop your friend from tempting you. If she keeps it up, see if you can find some written material that might get through to her. Your health care provider may have some suggestions. Or take your friend to a diabetes support group meeting where she is sure to hear that your feelings about being tempted are shared by other people who have diabetes.

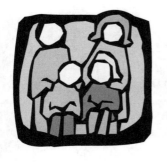

I have type 2 diabetes and I worry about other family members getting it. Is there any way it can be prevented?

TIP:

The short answer is yes. A recent study was conducted using people who were overweight and had a condition called Impaired Glucose Tolerance (IGT), sometimes called pre-diabetes. People with IGT have high blood sugar levels but not high enough to be called diabetes. About half of all people with IGT eventually develop type 2 diabetes.

There were 3 groups. One group received coaching in a healthy lifestyle designed to help them lose weight. Their goal was to be active (for most, this meant walking) 30 minutes a day, 5 days a week, and to lose 7% of their weight and keep it off. The 2 other groups took pills. One group took a medication called metformin (Glucophage) and the other group took placebo pills that looked just like the metformin but had no active medication.

The results of the study were impressive. People in the group who made lifestyle changes were 58% less likely to develop diabetes during the study than the people in the placebo medication group. Metformin also helped prevent diabetes during this study, but it was only half as effective as lifestyle changes. So, yes, it is possible to prevent diabetes, though we don't know for how long.

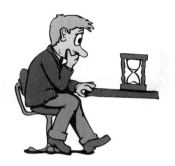

I've been waiting for a diabetes cure for years. When will it come?

▼
TIP:

That depends on what you mean by a cure. Pretty soon we should see some new tools that make it much easier to keep blood glucose levels closer to normal throughout the day. This wouldn't be a true cure, but it would help people with diabetes lead better, healthier lives. Along with better pills, better insulins, and better devices for delivering insulin, we could soon have glucose monitors that could be implanted in your body. Connecting an implanted glucose monitor to an insulin pump would create an artificial pancreas, which could do almost as good a job as a real pancreas.

A true cure for diabetes is still some years away. To cure diabetes we need to solve the two problems that cause diabetes: insulin resistance (problems using insulin effectively), and destruction of the beta cells that make insulin. People with type 2 diabetes have both problems, while people who have type 1 diabetes have problems only with beta cell destruction. We don't yet have a cure for diabetes, but we have made a lot of progress toward this goal in the past few years. You may see the day when diabetes is a disease of the past.

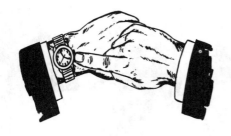

My blood sugars seem to shift by the minute but I can't check my blood that often. I've heard it is possible to monitor blood glucose levels continuously. Is this true?

TIP:

Several companies have developed continuous glucose measuring systems. One such device is the GlucoWatch Biographer, which is worn like a watch and measures glucose under the skin. It displays readings every 20 minutes for 12 hours, and stores up to 4,000 readings. The GlucoWatch can be programmed to signal if glucose levels rise above or fall below preset levels, or if glucose levels fall rapidly. You still have to check your glucose the old-fashioned way every 12 hours to calibrate the device, and the readings represent what your glucose level was 15 minutes before, so they're not exactly current. For more information, go to *www. glucowatch.com.*

Another company has developed the Continuous Glucose Monitoring System (CGMS). The CGMS is currently available by prescription and is mostly used short-term to help people adjust insulin doses. A sensor is placed just under the skin and attached to a monitor, which is worn on your belt or carried in your pocket. The sensor records glucose levels every 5 minutes and is usually worn for up to 3 days. When the test is complete, the health care provider downloads data from the monitor into a computer. These data show when the person is high and low, and what insulin adjustments would help. For more information, go to *www.minimed.com.*

I use my computer to get a lot of diabetes information because it's so easy. Is the information about diabetes on the Internet reliable?

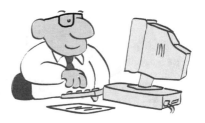

Not always. Though there is an amazing amount of valuable information on the Internet, a good portion of it is bunk. Along with lots of valid and helpful information, you will also find personal experiences that don't apply to you and outrageous claims designed to sell you a product. Separating the good from the bad can be difficult. The American Diabetes Association (*www. diabetes.org*) and the American Association of Diabetes Educators (*www.aadenet.org*) are good places to start when you want information, because they sponsor reliable sites. Many other organizations also sponsor websites featuring the latest diabetes research and other helpful information. There are also chat rooms where you can "talk" to other people who have diabetes and share experiences. You can learn a lot in a chat room, but keep in mind that you are hearing peoples' personal experiences, and these experiences might not apply to you. Before you act on something you see on the Internet concerning your diabetes, talk with your health care team to be sure it is right for you.

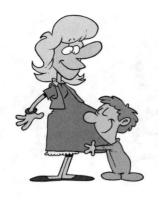

If I had gestational diabetes when I was pregnant will I get type 2 diabetes?

Not necessarily, but your risk does go up. The fact you had diabetes when you were pregnant means your pancreas has trouble keeping up with your insulin needs. About half of all women who have gestational diabetes will eventually develop type 2 diabetes. But there are things you can do to cut that risk. Studies show that if you change your lifestyle by eating more carefully, increasing your activity level, and losing weight, your risk of developing type 2 diabetes goes way down.

Changing your lifestyle is hard, but these changes are the same ones you should make if you get diabetes. Making those changes now could protect you from ever developing diabetes. Talk with your health care provider to learn more about your risk of getting diabetes and how to avoid it.

Chapter 9
DEALING WITH EMERGENCIES, TRAVEL, AND ILLNESS

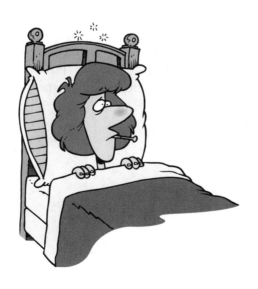

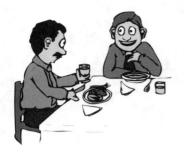

What should I do if I forget to bring my insulin when I go out to eat at a restaurant?

▼
TIP:

Things like this happen sometimes. If you can't go back to get your insulin, you have a few options to help minimize the potential negative impact on your glucose.

- Select foods that have less impact on your glucose level. Carbs have the biggest impact, so try to steer clear of those.
- Eat less of what you order. You can almost always take home the remaining food for a tasty snack when you are better prepared to deal with it!
- Exercise after the meal. Try taking a brisk walk.
- Take a shot of rapid acting insulin as soon as you can after the meal. If you choose this strategy, make sure that you check your blood glucose before and an hour or so after you take the insulin. Also, don't overcompensate; it is better to be conservative.

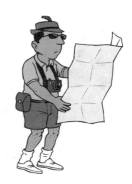

When I travel I'm always afraid I'm going to forget something. What diabetes supplies should I take when I'm away from home?

▼
TIP:

Pack twice as much of everything you would normally need if you were at home. This includes:

- Blood glucose monitor and strips
- Medication
- Syringes or pump supplies if you use insulin
- Ketone testing strips
- A source of fast acting carbohydrate (in case you experience a low blood sugar)
- If you are traveling during a mealtime, enough food to cover that meal

Extra food is a good idea in case you get stranded at an airport or your car breaks down. If you have to go through airport or border security, a letter from your doctor explaining why you carry syringes can be helpful. Check with the American Diabetes Association website (*www.diabetes.org*) for current recommendations for travel.

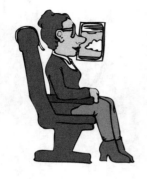

I'm never sure how to adjust my insulin when I travel. What adjustments should I make when I cross time zones?

▼
TIP:

This depends on your insulin regimen, where you are going, and how long you will be gone. We'll assume you use either an insulin pump or a combination of long acting and rapid insulin injections. If it's a short trip across one or two time zones, it might be best to take your basal insulin (basal rate for pump or long acting insulin by injection) at the same hour of the day in the time zone that you usually take your insulin back home. For instance, if you live in Kansas and you're visiting New York, where it's an hour ahead, take a 9:00 A.M. basal at 10:00 A.M. Then, simply take your boluses or mealtime shots of rapid acting insulin when you eat.

Another option is to continue taking your basal insulin at the same time you would at home, without taking into account the time difference. This means less adjustment, but you might end up with problems controlling your glucose if there is a big time difference. If you try this approach, check your glucose frequently. You may have to make adjustments with your rapid acting insulin to help keep your glucose levels close to normal.

I'm feeling stressed about traveling by plane with my insulin and syringes, especially since September 11. What should I do?

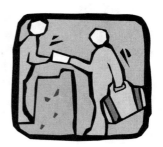

▼
TIP:

You do **not** need a prescription for your insulin or syringes. You simply need proof that what you are carrying is insulin. For proof, the Federal Aviation Administration (FAA) says you should keep the box that your insulin came in (or the plastic bag your boxes came in, if your insulin came from a mail-order pharmacy). These packages should have the information the FAA requires—"a professional, pharmaceutical pre-printed label which clearly identifies the medication." So don't throw away the original box or bag for your insulin if you plan to travel by plane. You can also carry lancets on the plane, as long as they are capped and you are also carrying "a glucose meter that has the manufacturer's name embossed on the meter."

Since September 11, 2001, the FAA has issued new security measures that apply to people with diabetes. Each airline might enforce these measures slightly differently, so it is best to check with your airline before traveling. You can also go to the ADA website (*www.diabetes.org*) for the latest guidelines. More than likely, you won't have any problems. But like always, it is best to be prepared.

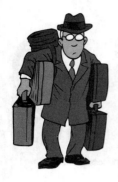

*I'm afraid my insulin pump will set off
alarms in airports. Is this possible?*

Reports vary. Some detectors may be more sensitive than others. Some people say their pump always sets off the alarm, others say that it occasionally sets it off, and still others say it never does. Insulin pumps are made mostly of plastic, so even if you do set off an alarm, your pump might not be the cause. If you are carrying or wearing anything else that could have triggered the alarm, you could remove or point out those things first. If there are no other potential causes or the security guards ask to search you, tell them that you have diabetes and you are wearing a medical device that delivers insulin. Offer to show them the pump and how it works. Carry a letter from your doctor saying (as simply as possible) that you need the pump and how the pump works.

As always, when it comes to coping with diabetes, a little planning and a little common sense will take you a long way.

*W*hy *is it so much harder to control my blood glucose when I am sick?*

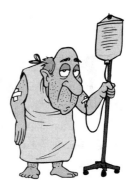

▼
TIP:

Being sick stresses your body, and stress can raise your blood glucose. Any kind of stress—physical or mental—can have that effect. So when you are sick, you have to take extra precautions to be sure your blood glucose doesn't go too high.

It's hard when you are not feeling well, but when you are sick you need to monitor more closely. The ADA recommends that you check your blood glucose and urine ketone levels every 4 hours. If your blood glucose level is high, it's a sign you need more insulin. If your urine ketones are 3+ or higher, it's a sign you need more insulin and probably some fast acting carbohydrate like regular soda, as well.

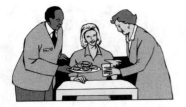

*W*hat are the best foods to eat
when I am sick?

▼
TIP:

S ince you need to stick to your regular diabetes medication when
you are sick, it's important to eat something, even when you
can't eat regular food. Most people find that things like regular soda,
fruit juice, sherbet, frozen juice bars, pudding, applesauce, and ice
cream are the easiest to eat, but anything with calories that you can
keep down will do.

Dehydration is a real risk if your blood glucose stays high for a
long period of time. So fluids like soda and juice are especially good
when you are sick because they help protect you from dehydration.
Broth and vegetable juices are also good because they help replace
the minerals you lose through vomiting and diarrhea.

A^{t what point should I call my doctor}
when I am sick?

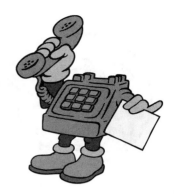

▼
TIP:

Your doctor is the best person to answer this question. Be sure to talk with him or her to see if the guidelines we discuss below apply to you. Generally, here are some things that should probably prompt you to call your doctor when you are sick:

- Not being able to hold down fluids. If you go more than 12 hours without being able to hold down fluids, you are probably getting dehydrated and you could get really sick without proper care.
- High urine ketone levels. Urine ketone levels that stay at 3+ or higher are another source of potentially serious problems.

Hopefully, you will rarely get so sick you need to call your doctor. But it is good to know the signs that signal you need help, so you will know when to make that call.

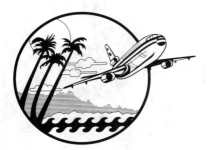

*W*hy *is it so hard to control my
diabetes when I travel?*

▼
TIP:

Travel often throws your diabetes management plan for a loop. Everything changes—you eat all your meals in restaurants, your activity level is probably changed and inconsistent, and unexpected stresses that push up your glucose levels lurk everywhere

Here are some suggestions for making good control a little easier when you travel.

- At restaurants, ask about the ingredients of the menu items so that you can avoid post-meal highs or lows.
- Frequent blood glucose monitoring can help you catch potential problems early, thus preventing highs and avoiding lows.
- Travel with workout clothing. Most hotels have exercise facilities and you can ask the hotel staff about safe places to walk outside the hotel.
- Always wear comfortable shoes when you travel so that you can walk briskly at every opportunity.

INDEX

▼

About the American Diabetes Association

The American Diabetes Association is the nation's leading voluntary health organization supporting diabetes research, information, and advocacy. Its mission is to prevent and cure diabetes and to improve the lives of all people affected by diabetes. The American Diabetes Association is the leading publisher of comprehensive diabetes information. Its huge library of practical and authoritative books for people with diabetes covers every aspect of self-care—cooking and nutrition, fitness, weight control, medications, complications, emotional issues, and general self-care.

To order American Diabetes Association books: Call 1-800-232-6733. http://store.diabetes.org [Note: there is no need to use **www** when typing this particular Web address]

To join the American Diabetes Association: Call 1-800-806-7801. www.diabetes.org/membership

For more information about diabetes or ADA programs and services: Call 1-800-342-2383. E-mail: Customerservice@diabetes.org www.diabetes.org

To locate an ADA/NCQA Recognized Provider of quality diabetes care in your area: www.ncqa.org/dprp/

To find an ADA Recognized Education Program in your area: Call 1-888-232-0822. www.diabetes.org/recognition/education.asp

To join the fight to increase funding for diabetes research, end discrimination, and improve insurance coverage: Call 1-800-342-2383. www.diabetes.org/advocacy

To find out how you can get involved with the programs in your community: Call 1-800-342-2383. See below for program Web addresses.

- *American Diabetes Month:* Educational activities aimed at those diagnosed with diabetes—month of November. www.diabetes.org/ADM
- *American Diabetes Alert:* Annual public awareness campaign to find the undiagnosed—held the fourth Tuesday in March. www.diabetes.org/alert
- *The Diabetes Assistance & Resources Program (DAR):* diabetes awareness program targeted to the Latino community. www.diabetes.org/DAR
- *African American Program:* diabetes awareness program targeted to the African American community. www.diabetes.org/africanamerican
- *Awakening the Spirit: Pathways to Diabetes Prevention & Control:* diabetes awareness program targeted to the Native American community. www.diabetes.org/awakening

To find out about an important research project regarding type 2 diabetes: www.diabetes.org/ada/research.asp

To obtain information on making a planned gift or charitable bequest: Call 1-888-700-7029. www.diabetes.org/ada/plan.asp

To make a donation or memorial contribution: Call 1-800-342-2383. www.diabetes.org/ada/cont.asp